Profe
Break the ~~Chains of~~ Smoking

"Todd Goodwin, in his new book *Break The Chains Of Smoking,* has written a clear, concise method to help people break this deadly habit. From attitude to action, he shows the light of hope. He also gives the obstacles that stop most people. He also give tips, research and client testimonials to inspire and give more power to the change. This book is a must read for anyone wanting to change this behavior. The only problem I have with this book is I didn't write it."

– William D. Horton, PsyD, MCAP
Psychologist, world's top NLP & hypnosis trainer, and author of *The Alcohol and Addiction Solution* and *Neuro-Plasticity and Addictions: New Pathways for Recovery*

"*Break the Chains of Smoking* is an informative, powerful, kick-in-the-pants kind of book that will help smokers get out of their physical and emotional prison. Todd Goodwin has tremendous depth of knowledge in this area, and shows us the emotional traps that keep people stuck, as well as how to escape those traps. His book is full of wisdom, humor, and reminds the reader that they hold the power to their success. A must read for someone who is ready to stop smoking."

– Judi Woolger, MD, FACP
Board Certified Internist and Chief Medical Officer, The Agatson Center

"*Break the Chains of Smoking* is inspiration in a book. Smokers who are truly ready to quit and have failed in all other attempts will finally get the breath of fresh air they are looking for. Todd understands why people end up feeling like a slave to cigarettes and gives them a clear path to freedom."

– Sandra Doman, DC
Chiropractor and founder, Miami Sports Chiropractic & Yoga Center

"I am delighted to see that hypnotist Todd Goodwin has put his ideas and experiences into a book. Smoking is a powerful addiction and so difficult to break for too many people. He provides an overview of the disease and a well thought out plan on how to help you recover. This book is a must read for anyone suffering from smoking addiction or wanting to understand more about the disease and its treatment."

– Eva Ritvo, MD
Psychiatrist, author, and founder, Bekindr Global Initiative

"Todd Goodwin has hit the nail on the head, as it is the mind and its beliefs that need to be dehypnotized and heal. Unless that is done, other methods are futile. He has developed a whole program to help the mind heal its old beliefs."

– Kirby R. Hotchner, DO
Osteopathic Physician, practitioner of holistic and integrative medicine, and founder, The Wholeness Center

"I have known Todd Goodwin and have referred patients to him for many years. I have learned to pay attention to what he says and writes. *Break the Chains of Smoking* cuts to the chase and gives clear instructions and support on how to finally break the habit. By exploring the true mind-body connection and the realization that smoking is primarily an emotionally compulsive habit, Todd explains how to get to the root of the problem. His clearly defined points to address the emotional and physical elements of quitting cigarettes are relatable. In addition, Todd gives you to the option to add another tool to your toolbox with the support of his online hypnosis system. If you want success in this journey, I highly recommend this book as a guide that will resonate with issues that have prevented you from breaking the chains of cigarettes in the past."

– Jane A. Kaufman, L.Ac
Board Certified Acupuncture Physician

"I read *Break the Chains of Smoking* with great interest and found, not only did it benefit my approach in assisting my own patients, but also discovered some facts about any addiction or habitual practice. Todd writes with a profound ability to engage the reader and leaves one with a desire to improve in whatever may be creating an addictive habit. In essence, I found the writing to be an approach for resolving the root cause of any person's need to use smoking for easing one's suffering, and with compassion observe the healing that may be required so smoking is no longer a self-sabotaging practice. With humor and kindness, as well as clear facts, Todd will guide anyone to become a better person and liberate themselves of the subconscious suffering by his proven methods of successful practice. I highly recommend this wise writing for anyone and everyone, not just for quitting smoking, but any habit that binds us. With great appreciation and respect, I thank you Todd for helping me on my own path."

– Kamran Khan, DOM, AP, DNBHE, C.Ht.
Doctor of Oriental Medicine and Homeopathic Diplomat

"As a Certified Hypnotist with my own practice, I work with many people attempting to quit smoking. As I have come to realize, smoking is an addiction that has very little to do with nicotine dependency. The roots and underlying causes of this harmful crutch are often deep and multilayered in the psyche and are a result of emotional dis-ease. Todd does an EXCELLENT job at explaining the nuance, difficulties, and particulars that often arise within each client attempting to quit. While practicing and seeing clients myself, this book often serves as a "manual" for many of the reminders and unique examples of the human experience with regard to smoking addiction, which aids in my knowledge and expertise. Whether you are assisting others to cease smoking or looking to quit yourself, this book is a MUST READ."

– Brad Plotkin, C.Ht.
Certified Hypnotist

"I have been around several smokers in my life including friends, family members, and patients at my holistic nutrition practice. I can confidently say that Todd's book, "Break the Chains of Smoking," is a clear and direct guide for reprogramming the mind and successfully breaking the terrible habit of smoking through the process of hypnosis. This book provides an easy understanding of how one may perceive the addiction and why it's useful to apply the effective remedy of hypnotherapy. It's a mind-opening read and I highly recommend it for anyone struggling with smoking or for anyone with loved ones who just can't quit."

– Galit S. Zarco, M.S., RD, LDN
Registered Dietitian, holistic nutritionist, and owner, Eat Live Nutrition

Break the Chains of Smoking

How to Escape the Mental and Emotional Prison That Keeps You Addicted

Todd Goodwin
Board Certified Hypnotist

Laughing Coyote Publishing
Sedona, Arizona

Break the Chains of Smoking: How to Escape the Mental and Emotional Prison That Keeps You Addicted

Published by Laughing Coyote Publishing, Sedona, Arizona

www.BreakTheChainsOfSmoking.com

ISBN-13: 978-1-7330707-0-6 (ebook)
ISBN-13: 978-1-7330707-1-3 (paperback)

First Edition May 2019

Trademark notice: Product or corporate names may be trademarks or registered trademarks of their respective owners and are used for identification or explanation without intent to infringe.

Disclaimer: The content contained within this book and the associated hypnosis programs are not intended in any way to diagnose, treat, heal, or cure medical conditions, illnesses, disorders, or diseases, nor are these products represented as any form of psychological, physical, or medical therapy, medical advice, or health care services. This material is held out to the public as a form of motivational coaching for self-help and educational purposes. Despite research to the contrary, we may make no health benefit claims for this content, which is intended to complement, not substitute for, any medical treatments, counseling, or therapy of any kind that may be appropriate for you. By following the recommendations offered in this book, and by using the hypnosis programs, you agree to accept any risks and release the author and any affiliated parties from any claims for liability that may result from doing so. Any and all results you achieve in the future are due to your own thoughts, beliefs, decisions, and actions, and you are fully responsible for those results.

"Addiction is the only prison where the locks are on the inside."

– Unknown

About the Author

Todd D. Goodwin, M.S., BCH, FNGH

Board Certified Hypnotist
Master Practitioner of NLP
Fellow, National Guild of Hypnotists

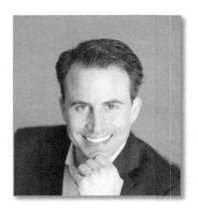

Todd Goodwin is in rare company as a Board Certified Fellow of the National Guild of Hypnotists, since only one in every 500 hypnotists have earned that designation. He is a certified master practitioner of neurolinguistic programming (NLP) and a member of the Academy of Integrative Health & Medicine. Todd has studied human behavior since 1995, earning a bachelor's degree in Behavioral Science from Washington University in St. Louis and a master's degree in Nutrition and Health Promotion from Simmons University in Boston. Since opening Goodwin Hypnosis (formerly the Miami Hypnosis Center) in 2007, Todd has helped thousands of clients to resolve a wide range of challenges, including stress, anxiety, trauma, smoking, and other unwanted habits.

Todd has been trained by several experts in hypnotism and human behavior, including Dr. John Demartini, originator of the transformational Demartini Method. As part of his rapid change work with clients, Todd also employs an innovative, multi-sensory version of Integral Eye Movement Therapy as a faster and more powerful alternative to EMDR with broader applications, including post-traumatic stress, compulsive habits and addictions, phobias, and thought-based problems like worrying.

Currently, Todd sees private clients primarily for the rapid resolution of emotional trauma and its emotional and behavioral consequences. His strategy is to identify and resolve the underlying causes of these personal issues, instead of merely treating their symptoms. Todd's mission is to help people develop a greater awareness of the relationship between their mind, body, health, and life experiences, so they can think, feel, and do better. Todd works with his wife, Gina, a Board Certified Hypnotist and expert in smoking cessation and trauma resolution.

Todd can be reached at www.GoodwinHypnosis.com.

Client Testimonials

"I was a pack a day smoker for 30+ years. I had unsuccessfully tried Nicorette, Chantix, etc. I quit between the first and second sessions without the usual stressed feeling of fighting constant urges to smoke. This was an amazing experience. I strongly endorse the program!"

– Laura Russo

"I was a very heavy smoker for 15 years and had tried to quit 3 times. Each time, I not only failed at quitting – I gained a lot of weight trying. When I went to Todd Goodwin for help, he assured me that he would not only help me quit smoking, but that I would enjoy the process and possibly even lose weight! And that is exactly what happened! He helped to increase my confidence, make quitting smoking fun and helped me reduce my temptations to overeat during the process. I am extremely proud to say I have been a non smoker for 9 months and have lost ten pounds!"

– Jennifer Zawadzki

"I tried so many different smoking cessation products and programs over the past years. These included gums, patches, and pills. Finally, I decided to try hypnotherapy. It changed my life. I used to smoke like a chimney and enjoyed it like anything else, and now I'm happy to finally say that I am a non-smoker."

– Pasquale Pisana

"I never thought I'd quit and it would be so easy! Not only did I quit smoking, but I gained more confidence in myself in the process. I tried everything in order to quit help lines, gum, patches and good old cold turkey but nothing worked and hypnosis was my last hope. I have no urges to smoke and proud to say I'm a non-smoker. Todd you're amazing!"

– Michelle Hageman

"I can honestly say that hypnosis has changed my life forever. I want to thank Todd for all of his help and for the peace and clarity that he helped me achieve. Nowadays, when I hear that someone has an issue of some sort I tell them - you need hypnosis! Quite frankly, I don't know how people live without it!"

– Peggy Classe

"I can't believe I suffered for 8 years and was able to so easily solve all of my issues within weeks. I cannot thank Todd enough!"

– Amanda Taylor

"I tried absolutely everything to quit smoking but it was impossible for me. At first I was a little skeptical about the idea of what it mean to be hypnotized, but I latter found out that it's just a relax state of mind in which positive suggestion can actually help you change your behavior in a subconscious level. Todd, Thanks for helping me quit smoking and saving me for this ugly discussing deadly habit."

– David Kohn

"After trying everything possible I came to the conclusion after a reading a book that this was my last hope. And ill forever be grateful to GOD for giving me the courage to make this choice its been 5 weeks and trust me I cant even explain whats going on in my life right now all I can say is wow, amazing, unbelievable, I can go on forever. But what I will say is thank you so much Dr. Goodwin from the button off my heart thank you, thank you, May god bless you."

– Randall Sanz

"I had been making promises to myself about quitting since 4 years ago when I began to smoke again after 6 years. My self-esteem suffered because I couldn't keep my promises. When I went to see Todd I was very fearful. Past experiences in which I went through torture attempting to quit haunted me. I'd felt very obsessed, nervous and full of cravings. Todd felt confident that with hypnosis and his support I was going to quit easily. Even though I'm a person who is hard to convince, I trusted Todd since the first day. He is a caring and enthusiastic professional. I was amazed at how easy quitting was! I'm so happy! My self-confidence has soar. Thank you so much Todd!"

– Maria

Contents

Introduction

> "Giving up smoking is the easiest thing to do.
> I've done it a thousand times."
>
> – Mark Twain

Millions of smokers and ex-smokers would agree with Twain's sarcastic comment, because it is easy to quit smoking...but to remain that way is considered one of the most challenging lifestyle changes.

Billions of dollars are spent annually on smoking cessation aids that, despite consistent claims to the contrary, may not improve long-term success rates and may all be equally ineffective. Recent observational studies have found that nearly all of the real-world effectiveness that was previously attributed to nicotine replacement and prescription drugs actually resulted from the behavioral counseling that accompanied those medications.[1,2] The clinical trials that were designed to demonstrate the drugs' efficacy incorporated behavioral counseling, yet less than 2% of smokers who use a pharmaceutical aid in the real world actually undergo such counseling. As a result, the trial results cannot be generalized to the population at large. At the same time, quitting cold turkey has a dismal 3-5% success rate per attempt,[3] and yet the vast majority of those who have successfully quit smoking over time did so without medication.[4,5] This means that abruptly quitting smoking with no other help eventually works for most people, but not until many attempts that span years of disappointment, wasted effort, weight gain, health problems, and tens of thousands of dollars spent on cigarettes.

There is a good reason why mainstream medical treatments for smoking cessation, addictions, obesity, anxiety, trauma, and many other emotional and behavioral conditions fail for most people. Until very recently, the prevailing view of modern medicine has been that we are highly complex physical systems that can be modified through chemical manipulation. While I mostly agree with this assessment as it pertains to our bodies alone (my nutrition experience supports this view, as we biochemically manipulate our bodies whenever we eat), this severely limited view is responsible for the failure of such medical interventions.

I know that we are far more than mere biochemical machines to be tinkered with by physicians and biochemists who cannot see the big picture. Only in the past couple of decades has conventional medicine begun to seriously consider the now accepted concept of the mind-body connection. Your mind has tremendous potential power to influence the biochemistry and physiology of your body and brain. You can realize that power, if only you could understand the mind's role in this interconnected relationship and were given the opportunity and tools to transcend limiting beliefs based on conventional wisdom. I intend to help you harness that power, as it is essential if you want to quit smoking easily and naturally.

My professional work, which now stands at the controversial frontiers of health and wellness, may be completely mainstream some years in the future. Until then, we must entertain the incomplete perspective of the biochemical model and determine how to best direct our emotions, behaviors, and health by modifying our thoughts and beliefs. That is the true work of a hypnotist.

Everyone knows that smoking and nicotine are considered highly addictive. Few, however, realize that it is the mental and emotional prison, constructed by the limiting beliefs and emotional dependency on smoking, which causes most of the struggle with smoking cessation. As a result, quitting is usually very difficult unless it's addressed as a mind-body challenge. If you approach the process from a purely physical perspective (a chemical addiction), your chances of success are much lower than if you realize that smoking is primarily an emotionally compulsive habit.

Most smokers' challenges are caused less by nicotine itself than by the beliefs that nicotine is highly addictive, that quitting smoking is difficult, and that many attempts, relapses, and withdrawal symptoms are likely before you ultimately succeed. These disempowering beliefs have been sold to the public by uninformed physicians with good intentions and by drug companies who profit from selling minimally effective smoking cessation aids.

Assuming that you really, truly want to quit, then your mind – if it's properly prepared, focused, and managed – is fully capable of eliminating cigarettes from your life forever, without relying on substitutes or suffering from withdrawal symptoms, and regardless of how much or how long you have smoked.

Since 2007, I've worked closely with hundreds of clients to help them quit smoking, so I know what does and doesn't work. I offer in this book what I believe to be the most essential insights related to quitting smoking. Much of what you will read is controversial because it challenges the prevailing societal view. Remember that society and scientists also once believed that the Sun orbited the Earth, germs didn't exist because we couldn't see them, and cigarettes were safe to smoke.

I have reviewed years of files from my smoking cessation clients and have identified which factors contributed to success and failure. If I were to adjust the success rate based on these factors, I would estimate that over 90% of my clients would have achieved lasting success if they had followed my instructions and applied everything that I will share with you. In other words, nearly all of their relapses or failures came from disregarding, or being unaware of, the lessons presented in this book.

As I will reveal, there are a number of factors that can determine whether you will succeed or struggle. The more you follow my recommendations, the more likely you are to succeed.

In fact, this is the first time that all these factors and insights have been compiled together, so you have a significant advantage over my past clients, since none of them had the full benefit of this material. While I cannot guarantee results, it is very likely that you will quit smoking for good IF you really want to quit, you take 100% responsibility for your actions and results, you make full use of this accumulated wisdom, and you use my online quit smoking hypnosis system. My confidence is enhanced by the fact that just 1% of those who have used my online program have asked for a refund under my money back guarantee.

As you read this book, you will come to realize that my hypnosis program will give you the greatest possible results for the smallest investment. While I have written this book with the expectation that you will take advantage of that opportunity, my recommendations will still be extremely useful even if you choose to rely on willpower, pharmaceuticals, or other methods.

A final thought before we get started. Please read (and re-read) this book with a very open mind, which means you must be willing to set aside the harmful and self-limiting beliefs you have accepted about smoking and quitting. It may be difficult and humbling to look in the mirror and realize that your lack of knowledge, excuses, and unresolved emotional issues have reinforced your toxic behavior. You, and everyone else who smokes, are fully responsible for creating, maintaining, and overcoming the habit, so if my commentary seems harsh at times, please understand that it's tough love, and that you need to hear it. You and I are both experts – you're an expert at smoking, and I'm an expert at quitting. The more you can accept my guidance – without beating yourself up – the better you will do.

Get ready to discover how to Break the Chains of Smoking, escape your mental and emotional prison, and quit smoking for the final time. You deserve it, and I know you can do it.

Part 1:
Open Your Eyes and See the Lies

"Don't bother me with facts, son. I've already made up my mind."

– Foghorn Leghorn

Confirmation bias is one of the most widespread and problematic biases of human thinking. It can be defined as the tendency to interpret new evidence as confirmation of one's beliefs and to reject new evidence that conflicts with those beliefs. During the past few decades, our society has been convinced by the medical community, pharmaceutical industry, and government agencies to believe that nicotine is the chief enemy in the battle against smoking. Once enough people fully embrace such beliefs (usually unknowingly), all new experiences and data points must pass through the filter of these beliefs. The incoming information is often rejected if it conflicts with the prevailing view, even when there is hard evidence that the established belief is incorrect. In other words, confirmation bias makes it more likely that we will defend what we already believe than be influenced by the facts.

The moment we accept the notion that some external opponent (nicotine, the government, the devil, etc.) is responsible for our problems, we become disempowered and are less likely to take responsibility for our own actions. Worse still, we will passively await a savior (a drug company, fast-talking politicians, God, etc.), rather than realizing how truly capable we are to save ourselves. You do possess that power and can make full use of it, only IF you can accept that truth, your desire is strong enough, and you are willing to persevere no matter what.

In this section, I debunk some of the most common rationalizations (rational-LIES-ations) and misunderstandings my clients have expressed upon first meeting me. It's very likely that you have thought or spoken some of these statements over the years. As you will come to realize, these are merely beliefs that seem very reasonable, but really just keep you trapped in the habit. Your beliefs influence your emotions, which then influence your behaviors. If you have limiting or disempowering beliefs, you will struggle and keep smoking. Once you realize the truth and change these beliefs, it is much easier to quit smoking and remain smoke-free. As you might expect, my hypnosis system helps to integrate a more useful and empowering belief system.

Here are 10 of the biggest "rational lies," in no particular order:

1. I'm a "smoker."

It's critical to understand that our identity ultimately dictates our behavior, so as long as you believe that you are a smoker, it will be very difficult to remain smoke-free. Most people spend at least as much time driving a car as they do smoking, and yet they don't define themselves as a driver.

Reality check: You've always been a non-smoker who's been trying to convince yourself to smoke. You were born as a non-smoker. The first time you had a cigarette, did you say, "Wow, this is delicious!" I highly doubt it. Unless you were drunk or high at the time, you probably coughed and thought it tasted awful. You then had to work very hard again and again to convince yourself to smoke (while choking) before you finally thought, "Wow, I can tolerate this," and you've been repeating that process ever since. This process of fixation, relaxation, and repetition is similar to hypnosis.

Therefore, if, like nearly every client I've seen who is honest with themselves, you also didn't like cigarettes at first, you can realize that you were a non-smoker who had to lie to yourself and light those cigarettes and choke them down many times before you learned to tolerate them. Basically, you hypnotized yourself into smoking, which means you need to be de-hypnotized. That's why hypnosis is an effective tool to quit smoking.

One important note: Throughout this book, I use the term "smoker" to refer to a person who smokes. Although using such a term is simpler for writing purposes, I strongly suggest that you disown that label as a self-identifier. Instead, consider yourself to be a non-smoker who, for many years until now, has chosen to smoke. Once you truly accept at the subconscious level that you are a non-smoker, it becomes easy to quit smoking and stay that way.

2. I'm chemically addicted.

It is a fact that nicotine affects brain chemistry by triggering reward centers in the brain.[6] It is fiction, however, that it controls your behavior. Even heroin addicts owe much of their problem to an emotional dependency, and cigarettes are vastly less dangerous or physically addicting than heroin. It's safe to say that most or nearly all of the smoking habit (and quitting smoking) is mental in nature – the habitual associations, the link to stress, and the belief that it's hard to quit. Several large studies suggest that the nicotine patch, gum, and lozenge fail over 90% of the time or produce results that are no better than using no cessation aid at all.[7-9] If quitting smoking were a simple matter of managing nicotine levels, then nicotine replacement therapy would be very effective. Modern medicine has no good options to sell to people who want to stop smoking, but it tries to convince you that it has.

Smoking is primarily a mental trap, so once you resolve the problem in your mind, nicotine becomes an irrelevant factor. Years ago, I learned of an Alzheimer's patient who woke up one day and actually forgot that he had smoked for 60 years. He had no withdrawal symptoms, no increased stress, and no cravings. In fact, he became disgusted and angry when he found what he believed to be someone else's cigarettes in his house. He proved that once your mind is able to relax its tight grip on smoking, just let it go, it's easy to stop. The only "addiction" of any real importance is the emotional dependency, which is based upon the belief that you need cigarettes. Emotionally compulsive habits can be broken once you address the emotions and underlying thoughts that cause them.

Here's another example to consider. Recall a time when you were running low on cigarettes, and when you reached for your pack, you found it empty. Or you were at home and thought you had a spare pack but couldn't find it. How did you feel? Many clients have told me that they felt stressed, anxious, or slightly panicky. When you went to a store to buy a pack or two, when did you first begin to feel better? Chances are, it was when you had the pack in your hand, or maybe after you left the store and pulled out a cigarette to light. Did the nicotine somehow magically make you feel better even before you took a puff? Of course not. You felt better because you had regained possession of something you had lost and mistakenly believed that you needed. If you believe that you need cigarettes to be okay, then it makes perfect sense to feel stressed when you are without them. Essentially, your control issues, more than nicotine, make quitting smoking difficult.

As soon as you realize that nicotine is a minor player, especially once you address its physiological influence (more on this later), you'll stop giving it credit and realize that you are in control. More importantly, once your subconscious mind adopts the belief that you don't need cigarettes or smoking at all, there are no cravings or difficulty quitting.

3. I'm going to have really bad cravings.

Many people are concerned about cravings after they quit. Truthfully, fear is the main reason that people who want to quit smoking fail to do so. Often it is the fear of cravings, which I distinguish from nicotine withdrawal. What is a cigarette craving? It is simply an urge to smoke, based entirely on emotional discomfort that can also manifest physically.

Your subconscious mind has been trained for years to remind you to smoke in many environments, situations, and emotional states. These reminders can continue for a time after quitting smoking (especially if you are not using hypnosis), and resisting these suggestions to smoke can create a stressful internal conflict.

What I find fascinating is that the urge to smoke is very similar to peer pressure. Your subconscious tells you to smoke, because the meal has just ended, or you're drinking alcohol, or you're driving, or you're with your smoking buddies. Resisting that insistent voice that repeatedly tells you to smoke can be especially difficult for people who gave in to peer pressure as teenagers. "Just have one. It will make you feel good. Don't let 'them' tell you what to do. You can do what you want." These are common messages that adolescents hear from their smoking peers as they have their first cigarette, and they are similar to what you may hear from your internal voice.

When the adolescent (and later, adult) learns that smoking alleviates or distracts from emotional discomfort, he or she relies on it to do so more and more. Whenever life presents an uncomfortable situation, however minor, smoking automatically becomes the preferred solution, however temporary it may be. As a result, the smoker rarely has to deal with the situation in an emotionally mature way, without the aid of a behavioral or chemical crutch. Essentially, people who developed the habit of smoking were emotionally immature, weak-minded, and easy to persuade when they first started, and that weak-mindedness and immaturity persisted for years as long as they gave in to the craving, urge, or subconscious reminder to smoke. Suddenly removing the crutch without building up emotional resources usually leads to elevated stress reactions, cravings, and habit substitution. Such responses are similar to those from frustrated teenagers who don't get what they want.

It's also ironic that most people started smoking because it was "cool," and yet smoking today is anti-social and anything but cool. The only way to be socially accepted again is to quit. Making a clear and powerful decision to stop smoking reveals a potential mental strength and emotional maturity that can support making this beneficial lifestyle change permanent.

If you recall how it felt to end an unhealthy or toxic relationship with someone and move on to improve your situation, you remember that it's something you used to know, but now it's behind you. You probably thought about that person occasionally for a while, but that didn't mean you wanted to go back to them, right? It's the same with smoking.

It's perfectly normal to think about cigarettes and smoking for a time after you quit, since you had a consistent relationship with that behavior for a long time. A passing thought about smoking is not the same as a craving or urge. Once you no longer want cigarettes at a subconscious level, there can be no cigarette cravings.

4. Cigarettes are like my friend.

If you have ever used the excuse, "It's like a friend, it's always been there for me," then you need some new friends. I've always thought that the comparison between a pack of cigarettes and a friend was pathetic. Your shoes have always been there for you, and you don't consider them to be your friends. You also don't feel bad about wearing them out and throwing them away. Shoes were designed to be worn and replaced, and cigarettes were designed to control you and keep you trapped.

Imagine a real person who tells you every day what to do and when to do it, who controls your social activities, who makes you waste thousands of dollars on him annually, who makes you stink so others judge or reject you, and who makes you look like an irresponsible fool when you're with him. You might claim that the two of you occasionally share good times, and you have some enjoyable memories with him from years ago. It's true that he helps to distract you from stress at times, but he does it just to keep you from leaving him. He steals your energy, he controls your daily schedule, and he harms your productivity. He causes your skin to age prematurely, he damages your gums and throat, and he also gives you coughs, colds, and lung problems. He makes you feel anxious when he's not around. Even after you break up with him, he persuades you to take him back again and again, so you lose integrity and feel powerless. If you remain friends long enough, he will share the gift of cardiovascular disease, COPD, cancer, or diabetes. He is your master, and you are his obedient slave…at least until you end this relationship.

Let's get real. Would you ever tolerate a "friend" like that in your life? You would need to have extremely low self-worth to do so. Sadly, I've found over the years that smokers, all else being equal, seem to have less self-worth and self-respect than non-smokers. That low self-worth is both a cause and effect of the smoking habit. It reminds me of a battered spouse who chooses to remain in a relationship with an abusive and controlling partner, because she's afraid to leave and rationalizes why it's acceptable to stay. Do yourself a favor and recognize that cigarettes are your greatest enemy, simply posing as a friend. Get a divorce from this toxic "friend" and move on.

5. It's hard to quit smoking. I lack the willpower needed to quit.

This statement is partially true, in that you likely do lack the willpower to quit. Fortunately, you don't need much willpower. Also, it's primarily your subconscious belief system that determines whether or not it's hard to quit, and it's up to you to change that. Your subconscious mind governs your drive to smoke, while your relatively weak conscious mind governs willpower. So your subconscious is the part that must agree to stop smoking for you to quit easily and permanently. Otherwise, quitting smoking can be extremely challenging and is usually temporary.

Willpower can be effective, such as refusing to see the dessert menu or ignoring a breadbasket at a restaurant, but it's a short-term solution. Interestingly, research has found that the more you rely on willpower, the more you deplete it, at least over the span of hours or days.[10] Willpower is also weakened with stress, fatigue, hunger, and low blood sugar.[11,12] As a result, most people do lack the willpower to change their habits, so relying on willpower to do so is difficult at best and pointless at worst.

Consider cold turkey. The 95+% of people who fail with any given attempt are likely using willpower, and that's why they fail. The 3-5% who succeed have made a decision to quit at the subconscious level, so willpower is rarely needed. Unfortunately, some successful cold turkey attempts lead to residual psychological dependency or to habit substitution, such as overeating, so they're only partially successful. As a result, the proportion of smokers who escape unscathed may be smaller than the 3-5% figure implies. Post-cessation psychological dependency and habit substitution occur because the subconscious retains its limiting beliefs about smoking, and its immediate need to ease discomfort still conflicts with the conscious, long-term goal to be healthy and free.

Once the two parts are integrated and in agreement, there is no increase in stress or eating after you quit. The bottom line is that forcing yourself to quit smoking, while certainly achievable, is unnecessarily difficult and can cause undesirable side effects like weight gain and elevated stress. So don't expect conscious willpower to solve your smoking problem. Focus on retraining your subconscious mind, and it will take care of the change for you.

6. I need to smoke because...

A common "rational-LIES-ation" is that you "need" to smoke, because you had a rough day, you're going through a stressful time, it helps you to focus, it prevents you from overeating, you get bad cravings whenever you attempt to quit, or your friends smoke. Although smoking is not a true need, it is rooted in the incorrect subconscious belief that you do, in fact, need to smoke. Our language is powerful and influences our thoughts, feelings, and actions, so it's important to be accurate. The more accurate and honest statement is, "I believe that I need to smoke."

In reality, there are hidden reasons that you may perceive your days to be rough, why you have trouble focusing, why you may tend to overeat, and why you experience cravings, and all of these issues stem from beliefs and conditioning you have reinforced over time. By changing at the subconscious level your thought patterns and their emotional consequences, you can resolve those factors that support your imaginary need.

Here's a tip. If you believe that you need to smoke in order to relax, note that much of the relaxation effect comes from detaching from what stresses you for a few minutes to breathe deeply. If you're willing to do the same thing without a cigarette, you'll love the breathing exercises in my online system.

7. Smoking doesn't serve any good purpose.

All behaviors begin with a positive intention or provide some benefit, even one as disgusting, harmful, expensive, and anti-social as smoking. People smoke because doing so helps them to relieve emotional discomfort or feel better. It's really that simple. If smoking didn't provide a benefit, even only occasionally, you would have already quit. There are many benefits, even if they don't justify the substantial costs to your emotional, physical, social, and financial wellbeing.

Honestly consider...Specifically how did smoking benefit you? What if you could get those benefits without cigarettes? My goal, as it is with all of my smoking cessation clients, is to help you find other ways (mostly at a subconscious level) to receive the benefits that smoking used to provide, and for you to learn to be comfortable smoke-free.

8. I must be an idiot to keep smoking.

It's easy to assume that you must be an idiot to continue to smoke, given all of the obvious drawbacks. From a long-term perspective, there are so many reasons why it is very stupid to smoke. But from a short-term perspective, it can be smart to smoke, given the possible alternatives, such as becoming overwhelmed, losing your temper, overeating, or abusing other substances. Resolving this apparent internal conflict requires an understanding of how the mind works. Simply put, your rational conscious mind thinks long-term and is well aware of the financial and health costs of smoking. That's the part of you that led you to read this book. On the other hand, your emotional and irrational subconscious mind thinks short-term, so it's concerned mostly with the next few minutes or hours, not next month or ten years from now.

Popular culture has illustrated this dynamic as an angel (conscious) on one shoulder and a devil (subconscious) on the other, each giving you conflicting messages. The subconscious wants you to smoke, because it has learned that you seem to "need" it to deal with the many (often minor) challenges each day. You now realize that it is a mistaken belief that you need to smoke, but the belief still triggers unpleasant emotions when you resist your subconscious commands. Rather than considering your subconscious to be an enemy, it's helpful to think of it as a misguided friend with good intentions who gives you bad advice. It's not trying to harm you. On the contrary, from its immediate perspective, it wants you to feel better, regardless of the long-term consequences.

Years ago, I met a client who had come to believe that he must hate himself, given his continued smoking in the face of all of the massive harm it had caused in his life. The only benefits he could acknowledge were that smoking helped him to manage his temper and contain his anxiety. I asked him if it were possible that he actually loved himself so much that he chose to smoke to prevent overwhelm from anxiety or anger. After all, for him, his daily emotional challenges were significant and immediate, while the disadvantages of smoking were more long-term or gradual in nature. This eye-opening realization that he smoked not because he hated himself but because he loved himself had a powerful effect on him, and it made it easier to quit smoking with hypnosis and learn to love himself in healthier ways.

When you understand yourself, your self-respect and self-esteem increase, stress decreases, and behavioral change becomes easier. The key to successful smoking cessation is to bring about an integration of the conscious and subconscious minds. An excellent hypnotist can facilitate this "mental handshake" that will allow you to be single-minded in your decision to stop smoking for good.

9. I like how cigarettes taste.

Have you ever had scotch? It tastes like gasoline, unless you've already consumed several ounces. I've known business executives who enjoy drinking scotch that costs $25 per glass and act like it's a big deal to drink it. But they're really lying to themselves, because it tastes horrible, at least at first. Nearly every person I know who "enjoys" the taste of scotch agrees and says that it's an acquired taste. Many of these same people also truly enjoy the flavor of chicken soup, orange juice, or hot chocolate, and they would readily admit that the flavor of scotch could not possibly compete with those other liquids in terms of gustatory pleasure. The reality is that they don't like the taste of scotch nearly as much as they like how they feel after a few drinks and what drinking expensive scotch means to them. So it's really a mental and emotional state they're seeking, not the delicious flavor of scotch.

Likewise, smoking is an acquired taste, as nobody naturally likes the flavor of burnt, chemically-infused tobacco. And no one has a natural desire to smoke, but one learns to do so to meet the need to take a break, relax, connect with others, or distract from unpleasant thoughts. No honest smoker will swear that they truly like the taste. Besides, smokers have a poor sense of smell and taste, so they can't judge accurately.

10. It feels good to smoke. I enjoy smoking.

It's important to understand that you convinced yourself that it feels good to smoke. Because smoking alleviates your emotional (and sometimes physical) discomfort, you have mistakenly given credit to the cigarette for making you feel better. In reality, however, it's your dependency on cigarettes that makes you feel bad to begin with and prompts the need to do something to feel better. In other words, the behavior that temporarily relieves your pain is the very behavior that causes the pain to exist in the first place. For non-smokers, it obviously feels normal, not uncomfortable, to not smoke.

Herein lies one of the major mental traps of smoking, or what most people consider its addictive quality. It's also why many people who quit smoking on their own tend to eat more and gain weight, since they're merely finding another unhealthy way to alleviate their discomfort.

You might protest that you don't smoke just to relieve discomfort. I understand that objection and respectfully disagree. Even if your discomfort is minor and you're not consciously aware of it, your subconscious is aware of it and tells you to smoke. Even if you feel fine, the impulse to smoke arrives preemptively to prevent withdrawal symptoms before they occur, so you're still smoking to ease the anticipated discomfort.

It's similar to how an obese person may eat constantly throughout the day so that he never actually gets hungry, because he is eating preemptively. Sometimes, that behavior is caused by a subtle or hidden fear of feeling hungry. As we all know with fear, anticipating discomfort can be quite uncomfortable. It sounds complicated, and it's true.

Let's dig a little deeper with a simplistic analogy. Imagine a 5-point numerical scale ranging from -2 to +2. A non-smoker's normal is 0. When he feels slightly good, it's +1. Slightly bad is -1. When people first smoke, it's -2, because it feels awful. Smoking repeatedly leads to habituation, or a reduced reaction to a negative stimulus. So when they begin to smoke regularly, new smokers become accustomed to the toxic onslaught caused by each cigarette. Smoking's harmful effect on the nervous system and stress hormones, combined with the gradual erosion of self-respect that is common among smokers, actually lowers the "set point" for what they consider to be feeling "normal" and "good."

Smokers feel uncomfortable when they're not smoking, so the new normal is now -1, not 0. Deprivation from cigarettes causes a drop to -2, and smoking raises it to 0. That's a real improvement, relative to feeling negative, but it's still not good. They smoke just to feel normal.

A related lie that smokers tell themselves is, "I enjoy smoking." The truth is that you don't really enjoy smoking nearly as much as you enjoy doing whatever you do while you smoke, as long as you're somewhat relaxed. You would most likely enjoy doing that same thing if you didn't smoke and were relaxed – having a drink, talking on the phone, driving, socializing with others after a meal, or taking a work break.

Most of my clients who smoked a pack a day admitted that the vast majority of their daily cigarettes were not very satisfying at all, and only a few were truly enjoyable. Usually the enjoyable ones had been smoked when they were feeling -2, so the relative improvement to 0 made them perceive the cigarette as enjoyable. So if your "normal" set point is negative, then you would mistakenly believe that smoking makes you feel good or that you enjoy smoking, when it's really just reducing discomfort and improving your level to 0 (non-smoker normal).

This subtle shift in perception is a trick that smokers play on themselves without realizing it. Once you quit smoking mentally and not just physically, your baseline normal returns to 0, so you can feel good more easily and frequently than when you were stuck in the smoker's negative mental trap. Without exception, the clients I've helped to quit smoking feel much better, happier, healthier, and freer as non-smokers, often within a few days. You can too.

Part 2:
Key Factors That Influence Your Outcome

"Success is the sum of small efforts, repeated day in and day out."
– Robert Collier

In this section, I share the insights that I've gained from helping hundreds of clients to quit smoking. Much of this invaluable wisdom emerged by observing the difference between successful clients and those who struggled to quit smoking. As I mentioned in the Introduction, none of my clients ever had the benefit of this entire body of essential knowledge, so you have an opportunity to profit from years of their collective experience.

Become very familiar with the factors I describe in this section, because all of them will influence your outcome, and any one of them could be responsible for your success or struggle. Remember that quitting smoking is determined primarily by your mindset and actions, so the more you are willing and able to adopt my perspectives here, the more likely you are to succeed with ease and escape from your mental and emotional prison.

Attitude and Mindset

"If you really want to do something, you'll find a way.
If you don't, you'll find an excuse."

– Jim Rohn

You can make excuses, or you can make progress, not both.

As detailed in Part One, most smokers have long ago mastered the art of lying to themselves. They have learned to rationalize why they smoke, why it's hard to quit, why they're not ready to do so, why they need to smoke, why they enjoy it, etc. It takes a well-developed habit of denial to justify or maintain long-term consumption of a known toxic and cancer-causing product.

Out of all of my clients, smokers had the greatest tendency to make excuses, nearly all of which were complete nonsense. When they struggled and had a cigarette, they said, "I had a stressful day," "I had a few drinks," "I was hanging out with my friends who smoke," "I was too busy to listen to my hypnosis programs," "I found a leftover pack of cigarettes in the kitchen drawer," and so on.

To be successful at this endeavor, just as with any goal, you must develop a strong sense of personal accountability and ridicule the absurd tendency to make excuses. Quitting smoking is absolutely within your power and ability, and no one but you can stop you from becoming smoke-free. You can be your own best friend or worst enemy. It's really up to you to choose.

Never say, "I hope it works."

Hope is a mostly useless emotion that takes your power away and puts it into the hands of something else. It's perfectly fine to hope that it doesn't rain, or that your plane arrives on time, or that your favorite football team wins. While it's pointless to do so, since your hope has zero effect on the outcome, it's not harmful. But it can be harmful to hope that you quit smoking "this time," because doing so unconsciously gives away your power and assumes that God, the Universe, a medication, or some other external force is going to help you out. That's wonderful if it happens, but realize that you are 100% totally and completely in control of this outcome. Don't assume that some outside force is going to help you, and don't hope that you succeed. Make sure that it happens. This subtle attitude shift is so much more important than you now realize. If you want it badly enough and are committed to your goal, you can do it.

Don't "try" to quit smoking.

There is a very powerful scene in Star Wars: The Empire Strikes Back that illustrates this point perfectly. Yoda, the small, but powerful Jedi Master, is training Luke Skywalker to develop his mental strength in the use of The Force. Luke's spacecraft has become stuck in a swamp. After Luke practices levitating rocks using The Force, Yoda tells him to do the same with his ship and lift it from the swamp. Here's the dialogue:

Luke: We'll never get it out now.
Yoda: So certain are you? [Shakes his head disapprovingly] Always with you it cannot be done. Hear you nothing that I say?
Luke: Master, moving stones around is one thing. This is totally different!
Yoda: No! No different! Only different in your mind. You must unlearn what you have learned.
Luke: All right, I've give it a try.
Yoda: No! Try not. Do. Or do not. There is no try.

Luke then tries and fails to recover the ship. Yoda lowers his head in disappointment as the ship falls back beneath the surface.

Luke: I can't. It's too big.
Yoda: Size matters not. Look at me. Judge me by my size, do you? Hmm?
Luke: You want the impossible.

Yoda then demonstrates his mastery of The Force by effortlessly levitating the ship from the swamp and returning it to solid ground.

Luke: I don't believe it! [Astonished]
Yoda: That is why you fail.

The key lessons in this scene, adapted to smoking cessation, are:

1. Doubting yourself or being certain of your inability to quit smoking will sabotage you.
2. Some of what you have learned from past failures can be helpful, but the learned expectation that the process will be difficult, painful, or futile will get in your way.
3. Do not "try" to quit smoking. Just do it. Trying implies failure, often after much effort. Just keep moving towards the goal until you have succeeded. It is completely within your power to do it, so don't let anything real or imagined stop you.
4. The most important lesson relates to what you truly believe. If you believe, at the subconscious level, that you will fail, you will likely fail. If, on the other hand, you believe that you were and are designed to be a non-smoker, and that you are fully capable of quitting smoking, then you will probably succeed. What you claim to believe consciously is not important. It's what you believe deep down that determines your experience and outcome. That is where the real work must be done.

More nicotine does NOT mean more difficulty.

It's a misconception that the longer you have smoked, and the more you smoke, the harder it will be to quit. While this may be true for a fraction of smokers, it is mostly a falsehood spread by the medical community and makers of nicotine replacement products or cigarette substitutes.

Over the years, I've delivered many presentations to physician groups, during which I provided anecdotal evidence that moderate-heavy smokers can quit smoking more easily than light smokers. The doctors were surprised, because their education, as well as conventional wisdom, said that more nicotine and more years equaled more difficulty. If we consider only the physical or biochemical model, that would be true.

However, because quitting smoking is mostly mental in nature, the collective forces of motivation, decision, and clarity of thought are vastly more powerful than nicotine. I have seen clients who have smoked as many as three packs per day and as few as two cigarettes per day. In some ways, it's easier for heavy smokers to quit, and in some ways it's harder. Overall, I have seen no consistent evidence that heavy smokers have a more difficult time quitting than light smokers.

Indeed, I recall two clients early in my career whose surprising results first gave me this insight. One client smoked a cigarette in the morning and before bed, and she needed four sessions over two weeks to stop smoking completely. She struggled, despite very low nicotine intake and infrequent smoking behavior. Another client who was referred by a local hospital's smoking cessation program had smoked two packs a day for 40 years. He had probably consumed more nicotine than any other client I had seen to that point. He stopped smoking completely at his first of four hypnosis sessions. He experienced no withdrawal symptoms, no emotional struggle or elevated stress, and no increased eating (and he was already overweight) as of eight weeks from our final session.

It was easier for the heavy smoker to quit because he was very aware of the negative effects of smoking in his life, while the light smoker had experienced very few drawbacks from her habit. Most physicians would have incorrectly predicted the opposite outcome for each client. Imagine all of the patients who were convinced by these medical experts that quitting would be hard, simply because of their lifetime nicotine consumption. What a disservice.

Remember that the stronger your reasons for quitting, the more successful you will be, regardless of the amount of nicotine you have consumed.

Nicotine Withdrawal

"One believes things because one has been conditioned to believe them."

– Aldous Huxley

FEAR: False Evidence Appearing Real

Fear of nicotine withdrawal is a major reason why smokers procrastinate quitting smoking, and their inability to handle discomfort is a primary reason so many attempts fail within the first couple of days. Many people don't realize that the body eliminates all nicotine within 72 hours of the last cigarette and half of it within two hours.[13] This temporary hurdle explains why smoking cessation becomes easier after several days pass.

Smoking affects a number of physiological functions and states, including blood sugar regulation, caffeine metabolism, and hydration.[14-17] Many smokers skip meals, drink large amounts of caffeine, and are mildly dehydrated, each of which could cause uncomfortable symptoms were it not for the consistent consumption of nicotine.

As the table on the following page illustrates, most symptoms of nicotine withdrawal are identical to those of low blood sugar, caffeine overdose, and dehydration. Smokers blame their physical discomfort on nicotine withdrawal, as they are unaware of this surprising correlation. They don't realize that many, if not most, withdrawal symptoms are caused by the hidden symptoms of pre-existing poor eating habits,[18] and not only by the loss of nicotine itself. Unfortunately, their discomfort after a day or two without smoking often leads them to find that smoking a cigarette makes the symptoms go away, so they never discover the truth.

As a former nutritionist, I was surprised that I had been unaware of the hidden link between nicotine and these dietary factors, just like many physicians I know. Fortunately, I discovered the correlation early in my hypnotism career. There's a corrupt conflict of interest that explains our shared ignorance – government agencies that decide public health policy and create smoking cessation guidelines receive funding from companies who make nicotine replacement and prescription drugs, as do major quit support websites and organizations like the American Cancer Society,

American Lung Association, and American Heart Association. It's no surprise that they all recommend pharmaceutical aids with questionable effectiveness over no-medication options that may be more effective.[19] We may all be victims of a well-orchestrated misinformation campaign.

Table Withdrawal Symptoms: Mistaken Identity or Misinformation?[20-24]

Nicotine Withdrawal	Low Blood Sugar	Caffeine Overdose	Dehydration
Headaches	Headaches	Headaches	Headaches
Dizziness	Dizziness	Dizziness	Dizziness
Anxiety	Anxiety	Anxiety	
Sweating	Sweating	Sweating	
Irritability	Irritability	Irritability	Irritability
Fatigue	Fatigue		Fatigue
Increased appetite	Increased appetite		Appetite changes
Constipation		GI disturbances	Constipation
Mood swings	Mood swings		
Lack of focus	Lack of focus		Lack of focus
Tremors/shakiness	Tremors/shakiness		
Cravings	Cravings		
Nausea			Nausea
Insomnia		Insomnia	
Restlessness		Restlessness	

Low blood sugar

Most of my clients shared the habit of skipping breakfast or consuming only coffee and cigarettes. Especially when combined with caffeine, nicotine causes an immediate blood sugar spike and suppresses appetite.[25,26] As nicotine levels start to drop after an hour or so, blood sugar also declines and may soon undercut normal levels (hypoglycemia) due to elevated insulin levels, thereby producing sugar cravings.[27] Smokers typically interpret these signals as nicotine cravings and respond by smoking again, which eliminates the symptoms. Quitting smoking without improving one's diet can lead to a period of these unexpected blood sugar dips, a condition that may resolve itself after several days, as long as one hasn't developed severe insulin resistance.[28]

Studies have found that dextrose (sugar) tablets quickly decrease the desire to smoke in the initial period after quitting,[29] as well as reducing irritability, hunger, and withdrawal symptoms.[30] These tablets also improve post-quit abstinence rates more than nicotine patches.[31] You can maintain healthy blood sugar levels in the days after quitting by not skipping meals and by eating fruit as a snack. If you experience a sugar dip or a strong desire for sweets, drink three or four ounces of fruit juice, ideally on an empty stomach. At 50 calories per dose, this will not cause any weight gain, assuming you do it only as needed for a few days.

Caffeine overdose

Numerous research studies have shown that nicotine significantly increases the rate of caffeine metabolism, which means that smokers clear caffeine from their body much faster than non-smokers. The more one smokes, the faster caffeine is eliminated.[32,33] This effect is the primary reason that smokers consume much more caffeine than non-smokers. In fact, clinical research suggests that smokers require three to four times the caffeine dose as non-smokers to reach similar blood plasma caffeine levels.[34] In addition, other research has found that, among smokers, each additional cigarette is associated with an increase in coffee intake by 0.1 cups, which totals two cups of coffee per pack of cigarettes.[35] After one stops smoking, caffeine levels in the blood can more than double if caffeine intake is maintained at the same level.[36] Unless consumption decreases significantly, symptoms of caffeine overdose may arise.[37]

I have often suggested that my clients reduce their caffeine intake by half immediately after their last cigarette. This step is not critical if you smoke only a few cigarettes, but it becomes increasingly important as the number of cigarettes approaches 10. Note that I don't recommend completely eliminating caffeine initially, as doing so can cause severe headaches. If your goal is to eliminate caffeine as well, it's better to do that gradually over a few weeks, depending upon your intake level.

Dehydration

Many smokers suffer from chronic mild dehydration as a result of several factors. First, smoking involves breathing in hot, dry air and exhaling moist air, so the lungs lose water throughout the day.[38] Second, smokers typically drink less water than non-smokers, because they favor caffeinated or alcoholic beverages, which are diuretics (promoting urination).[39,40] Third, the body's constant effort to reduce the toxic load from smoking can result in excess fluid loss through the skin, intestines, and kidneys. The importance of supporting the detoxification process is enough reason to drink a lot of water in the weeks after you quit smoking.[41] Remember that nature's solution to pollution is dilution.

The bottom line

Now that you understand how nicotine tends to mask the symptoms of dehydration and excessive caffeine consumption, while simultaneously and artificially propping up blood sugar, you realize that the unpleasant consequences of these underlying conditions are revealed once nicotine is removed from the picture.

If most smokers were to manage their blood sugar more effectively, reduce their caffeine intake, and drink plenty of water, their physical experience of quitting smoking would be much easier. Furthermore, if they were to combine this knowledge with an effective hypnosis protocol, they might even enjoy the potentially empowering process of quitting smoking, as a number of my clients were surprised to tell me.

It's worth noting that many of my clients did not adjust these dietary factors upon quitting, either because they chose to disregard my suggestions, or I did not know at the time how to advise them. Nonetheless, most of those who changed nothing still reported little or no withdrawal symptoms, most likely because of the powerful "mind over matter" effect of their hypnosis sessions.

Rest assured that withdrawal symptoms are very unlikely if you follow the dietary suggestions, reduce your stress, and use hypnosis as your chosen method.

Taking Action

"Many of life's failures are people who did not realize
how close they were to success when they gave up."

– Thomas Edison

If you quit the program early, you won't quit smoking.

When using my online quit smoking hypnosis system, you simply must follow through and complete the entire program as instructed, whether or not the process is as easy as you expected. Over the years, one of my recurring disappointments has been when clients disappeared after the first or second session and did not attend their remaining sessions, even after they had paid in full. While some of these clients realized long-term success after just one session, they were the exception to the rule, as I learned from later communications. Many of the disappearing clients had quit smoking immediately at their first session but often relapsed soon thereafter. Others struggled after their first session and then gave up, never giving themselves a real chance.

Unfortunately, the majority of those clients who abandoned their program for any reason ultimately brought about their own failure, so they wasted their time and money. As I recall, very few blamed me for their poor results, since they know they didn't do the work. Instead, they blamed themselves and further eroded their already damaged self-esteem. Blame is wasted energy. It is much better to take responsibility.

Please remember, it is absolutely critical to complete the program as instructed, because repetition and reinforcement are keys to learning. A major shift is often only one day away. If you're going to start, make sure to finish, regardless of how easy or challenging it may be.

If you were an actual prisoner who managed to escape from your abusive jailer, would you run only a few miles and then give up? Of course not. You would keep moving, no matter what, until you had fully secured your freedom. That is exactly how you must consider your situation as you quit smoking. I can assure you that if you apply what you've learned here, you will dramatically increase your likelihood of successful, long-lasting freedom from smoking.

Waiting for a health scare to quit smoking is waiting too long.

Sadly, I recall a man who came to see me after being diagnosed with lung cancer. I told him I could help him stop smoking, but he waited to schedule his appointments. Several months later, before he ever began my smoking cessation program, his wife contacted me to tell me that he had died. If only he had been motivated to quit several years before his diagnosis, he might still be alive today.

If it takes a cancer diagnosis or a heart attack for someone to finally wake up and decide to stop smoking, then that person is clearly out of touch with the harmful disadvantages of smoking and otherwise unmotivated. While many people do manage to quit after a medical incident, the scare often serves only as a temporary solution. Even if they do quit permanently, habit substitution (most often overeating and weight gain) tends to occur, especially since they didn't decide to quit on their own terms. In my experience, people whose primary motivation for quitting smoking was to avoid health problems tended to be less successful than those with stronger reasons. If you have been spurred into action by a health scare, then it's still worthwhile and quite possible to quit successfully, but you must find other powerful motivators.

Finances

"Investing in yourself is the best investment you will ever make.
It will not only improve your life, it will improve
the lives of all those around you."

– Robin Sharma

Focus more on your goal than what you will pay to achieve it.

I have often heard people ask, even before we have met to discuss their goal of quitting smoking, "How much does it cost?" While it sounds like they are asking about the level of investment, they're really asking, "How much money am I going to have to gamble on another attempt to stop smoking?" Their question reveals the very common, learned expectation that they are likely to fail, and so they must be comfortable with the degree of financial risk they are taking. If they could be guaranteed success, what would that be worth to them financially? It would be worth much more than the $1777 that I most recently charged for my private, customized smoking cessation services. Most of my clients had spent more than that amount each year on cigarettes alone.

When you are preoccupied with the "cost" of self-improvement, especially when it is modest compared to the cost of your problem, you cannot also be focused on achieving the goal. To succeed, you must accept the financial investment, consider the likely return on investment, and then focus entirely on the steps that are required to reach your goal. To do otherwise is a waste of time, money, and energy.

Consider the true cost of your problem.

Very early in my career, I had a client who was an accountant that smoked a pack a day for 30 years or so. During our initial consultation, I asked him how much money he spent on smoking. He told me that he spent around $2,000 per year in cigarettes, "…but I'm sure there's more than that." We agreed to work together, and he quit smoking easily.

He then came back to see me months later to help with a phobia, and I remember seeing a huge smile on his face as he walked in. I asked if he was smiling because he hadn't smoked in several months, and he said, "Yes, but I also figured out the answer to your question about how much money I'd save per year as a non-smoker…$5,000!" I asked how that was possible if he smoked only a pack a day.

This proud accountant then handed me a printed spreadsheet with twenty-something rows of numbers that itemized all of his previous smoking-related costs and other expenses that had decreased since he quit. At the top of the list were cigarettes, followed by life insurance, health insurance, car insurance, homeowners insurance, dry cleaning, carpet cleaning, cologne, breath mints, mouthwash, cold medications, air freshener, alcoholic beverages, doctor visits, and a dozen more. Today, that figure would be a lot more than $5,000 per year.

He also told me that those were just his out-of-pocket costs. His productivity improved since he wasn't taking constant smoking breaks or thinking about smoking when he wasn't smoking. Smoking was no longer a factor in planning his day. He was healthier, he had fewer sick days from work, and he didn't worry so much about future health issues. As a result, his stress level was lower, and his self-respect was higher.

Of course, saving money is never a great motivator to quit smoking. I've had several older clients who had promised themselves decades ago that they would quit smoking when cigarettes reached $3 per pack, but they didn't do it. Then it was $4 per pack, then $5, etc.

According to a 2018 study by WalletHub, smoking costs the average American smoker an estimated $1.8 million in a lifetime (averaging $35,000 per year), and more than $2.8 million in some states (averaging $56,000 per year). These figures include cigarettes, insurance premiums, healthcare costs, lost income, and financial opportunity cost.[42]

How much does smoking truly cost you financially? Even if money doesn't motivate you, it pays to consider other ways to use that money that you used to waste on smoking. I remember a client who rewarded herself for quitting smoking by spending the same amount of money to get a massage every two weeks. What could you do for yourself?

Pay for it yourself.

Over the years, I learned that clients are much less likely to succeed when a family member pays for their program. In some cases, the paying family member wanted his or her relative to stop smoking more than the smoker did himself, which is a recipe for failure. Remember that your desire to quit smoking for yourself is absolutely essential to your success.

In most cases, the family member paid because he or she wanted to incentivize the smoker, but doing so actually removed some of the incentive. We are also more likely to value and respect something when we have invested our own money. Of course, this was much more of a factor with my private quit smoking sessions than it is with an online program at a small fraction of the price. Nonetheless, however relatively small the investment in my program is, it's essential that you pay for it yourself, so you have some skin in the game.

You're going to pay for it, so do the work.

Everyone has been guilty of buying a book and not reading or finishing it. You also likely know someone who bought an annual membership at a gym but stopped going after a month or two. Unfortunately, making the purchase gives us a sense of satisfaction that we're truly taking action, when the important action must follow the purchase. You don't deserve credit for joining a gym or buying a book unless you make use of it.

Likewise, purchasing my online hypnosis system doesn't qualify as "trying" to quit smoking. It counts only if you do the work that is necessary to succeed. If you internalize the material in this book, follow the steps I recommend, and make full use of the program, you will likely succeed. If you don't plan to give it 100%, don't even bother to buy it. While a book publisher or fitness club doesn't care at all if you follow through, I actually do. I measure my professional success more by the quality and quantity of testimonials submitted by successful clients than from sales alone.

Remember Yoda's advice: "Try not. Do or do not. There is no try."

Relationship Issues That Sabotage

"When the voice and vision on the inside becomes louder and more profound
than all opinions on the outside, you have begun to master your life."

– John Demartini

Unhealthy relationship patterns can present a real threat to otherwise promising cessation efforts. While many relationships may be supportive to the cause, my purpose here is to identify several potential pitfalls to watch for that can sabotage the partner who most wants to stop smoking. These relationship issues include codependency, competitiveness, resentment, and superiority.

For simplicity purposes, I use the term "spouse" and the most common examples of husband and wife. Note that these dynamics are not restricted to married couples, since other committed partners, family members, or friends can also interfere with the goal of successful smoking cessation. In general, there are three scenarios:

1. Both spouses smoke and try to stop smoking at the same time.
2. Both spouses smoke, but only one of them attempts to quit.
3. Only one spouse smokes.

Codependency

Let's address the first scenario and the potential problems that can arise. It's rare that both spouses are equally motivated to quit smoking at the same time. Usually one of them is more driven and committed than the other. Let's say that the wife is really serious about quitting, and the husband agrees to quit smoking to support her, so she is the leader, and he is the follower. In this type of situation, the husband typically fails, and witnessing his failed attempt can demotivate her. She may feel bad for her husband, especially if the two are codependent, not individuated from one another, or both too supportive of each other.

In other words, the actions or reactions of one spouse can significantly affect that of the other spouse, as though they are not each separate

31

individuals capable of following their own distinct path and making their own decisions.

Competitiveness

Competitiveness, which is a potential problem at the other end of the spectrum, can also occur when both spouses try to quit smoking together. Consider two competitive spouses who want to "beat" each other at the smoking cessation game. On the surface, this seems absurd, but it is usually completely unconscious and unintentional. Still, given the various forms of resentment that can develop in committed relationships, this competitive nature can bring about certain words or emotions in one spouse that trigger the other.

For example, each spouse may be passive aggressive, which can be a subtle form of hostility. If both parties are not acting in the best interest of the other, problems will arise. In both of the above cases, one spouse can manage to sabotage the other.

Resentment

Relationships can be threatened when one person grows while the other stagnates. In the second scenario identified above, let's assume that the wife wants to quit, but her husband does not. He may unknowingly resent her for trying to better herself, as though her success makes him inferior by comparison. Or he may feel as though her quitting smoking will harm their relationship, since they will no longer share smoking and everything it involves. If the husband's insecurities stem from resentment, he may act passive aggressively or be verbally hostile to her. This unsupportive behavior can lead to the wife (in this case) relapsing.

This dynamic is similar to how some of your smoking friends may unconsciously hope that you keep smoking, so you will still spend time with them. You can witness this phenomenon, known as "crabs in a bucket," by placing several live crabs in a bucket and watching as one crab nearly manages to escape. Often, one of the remaining crabs will reach up and pull the escaping crab back into the bucket. I don't claim that they're aware of their actions, but it's analogy you'll remember. Ask yourself which family members and friends share the bucket with you. Could they, selfishly, try to pull you back in once you start to escape?

Superiority

Similar challenges can arise with the third scenario, in which only one spouse smokes. Specifically, the non-smoking spouse makes comments that belittle the other and prompt him or her to resume smoking. I've heard many clients recall a family member say, "You've been in a bad mood since you quit. If this is how you're going to be, you should start smoking again." Or "I liked you better as a smoker."

Separately, the non-smoking spouse may act like he or she is superior to the smoking spouse and say, "See? I've always told you that you would feel better after you quit. You should listen to me, since I'm usually right." This attitude can evoke a parent-child dynamic and cause the spouse that smoked to rebel against the other spouse's assumed authority. As a result, the now ex-smoker's need to engage in the marital power struggle can lead to relapse. Remember, you can fight to be right or you can stop fighting and be happy. I recommend the latter.

Dealing with friends

There is an excellent strategy for dealing with your friends as you prepare to quit smoking. My clients and I have found that declaring your intentions and making a social commitment will improve your likelihood of success. That does not mean that you should tell everyone you know, since (as seen above) some people will not want you to change. Some of my past clients have taken the opposite approach and didn't tell anyone of their plans to quit. Their decision, based in fear that they would look bad or need to explain themselves if they failed, is a poor one, not because they would deprive themselves of social support, but because keeping the secret reinforces their own expectations of failure.

To successfully quit smoking, it's critical that you develop an expectation of success, since it's totally within your control. I suggest that you tell only those people whom you know will serve as your cheerleader and also hold you accountable for making excuses or slipping back into old behaviors.

It's also well established that we are greatly influenced by the people we spend the most time with. So if your friends routinely engage in unhealthy behaviors like smoking, then their influence is holding you back from living the better life that you deserve. Similarly, if your friends or family members tend to be very negative, complain about their problems, other people, or a lack of money, or otherwise pollute your environment with toxic words or energy, it's very likely affecting you.

My recommendation to clients who have expressed this concern has been to seek new friends whose attitude and lifestyle reflect how you want to be in the future, not how you were in the past. Over time, you will likely enjoy being with your new friends more than the old ones, since you'll have more in common with them. You don't have to dump your old friends, as they may find their way out of your life on their own.

Other Potential Pitfalls

"Rule your mind or it will rule you."

– Horace

Emotional stress

Stress is one of the most common triggers for smoking and causes of relapse.[43] If you don't manage your stress, you won't manage to quit. Since nearly all smoking is triggered by the short-term-oriented, subconscious drive to escape from discomfort, excess stress and an inability to handle stress usually interfere with quitting smoking. To address this potential challenge, my hypnosis system incorporates several aspects of stress reduction. First, the hypnosis programs themselves relieve stress, as the state of hypnosis triggers a relaxation response. Second, repeatedly accessing this relaxed state conditions your nervous system to relax more readily, so it becomes easier to relax throughout your day and at night. Third, much of the hypnotic language and program content is geared towards reducing stressful thoughts and increasing self-confidence. Fourth, the techniques I provide to rapidly trigger a relaxation response or clear your mind will be valuable tools during the smoking cessation program and will be useful long after you have quit smoking.

Low self-worth

Self-worth, defined simply, is how you value yourself. It's related to self-esteem, which is how much you like yourself. If you believe that you truly deserve to achieve your goal, it's much easier to do so. If, on the other hand, your self-worth is less than what you need to achieve a goal, you may unconsciously sabotage yourself to stay true to your self-image.

Consider someone in an unhealthy relationship whose friends say, "You can do so much better than that person. Don't you know you deserve to be with someone who appreciates and respects you?" I've had many (mostly female) clients who have trouble leaving partners who treat them poorly. One of the reasons they feel stuck is that they don't truly feel that they deserve a healthy relationship. They may understand rationally that they deserve better, but emotionally, based on childhood programming or past relationship experiences, they don't believe it.

Your relationship with smoking is essentially an abusive or controlling relationship, and I bet that your true self-worth is not as high as you might think, or you may have already quit smoking. Low self-worth can be caused by guilt related to a past experience or shame about some aspect of yourself that you have never accepted. Shame (and its resulting low self-esteem and anxiety) is a major reason why the incidence of cigarette smoking is 42% higher in the LGBT community than among heterosexuals, according to the CDC.[44] Growing up while feeling rejected by a parent can also cause a lack of self-worth that can produce chronic stress or anxiety. If our self-worth depends upon others' approval or love, we become more susceptible to toxic relationships, as well as behavioral problems like smoking, alcohol abuse, and overeating.

Ask yourself if you feel, even slightly, that you don't deserve to be a healthy non-smoker, and contemplate how your own self-judgments have helped you to draw that erroneous conclusion.

Low self-efficacy

Henry Ford said, "Whether you think you can or you think you can't, you're right." Self-efficacy is your belief that you can create change in your life or achieve goals. If you have high self-efficacy with respect to smoking cessation, you believe that you absolutely can quit smoking. If you have low self-efficacy, then you don't believe it's going to happen, even if you have high self-worth. In this case, believing that you lack an effective action plan, sufficient emotional resources, social support, or perseverance will result in a loss of motivation to take consistent action.

Among smokers, low self-efficacy is very common and responsible for the relative infrequency of quit attempts. After all, if 68% of smokers want to quit smoking,[45] why would only 28% attempt to quit over a period of three years?[46] Reading this book should give you the confidence that it's very achievable for you to stop smoking for good. Furthermore, these recommendations, combined with my online hypnosis system, provide a powerfully effective action plan.

Consider the many tasks or goals you have accomplished that are truly more difficult than quitting smoking, and your self-efficacy will increase. Once you are smoke-free, you'll look back and realize that smoking cessation was much easier than most of those other achievements.

Secondary gain

We can define secondary gain as the benefit provided by the problem state. This fascinating phenomenon explains why people often sabotage their health, relationship, and financial goals, especially after they have made some progress. It can explain why someone might really want to stop smoking but relapse repeatedly after having successfully quit for a period of time. It can also explain why someone would start using a quit smoking hypnosis system, realize great results, and then stop using the program before it's complete. This would be like escaping from prison and then later deciding to turn back and return to the jail cell.

Another explanation of secondary gain is a situation in which it is apparently better to remain stuck with a problem than to solve it, and when the solution presents new problems that may seem greater than the current problem. In effect, the subconscious mind reestablishes the problem for self-protection, despite the obvious disadvantages of keeping the problem.

In fact, many people with ongoing issues like obesity, chronic pain, and grief are actually receiving a hidden benefit so great that they subconsciously (unintentionally) avoid or resist solving those problems. The secondary gain or benefit is usually emotional support, avoidance of a perceived challenge, or both.[47] While this phenomenon does not always play an obvious role in smoking, there are potential disadvantages of quitting smoking, including loss of relationships or weight gain. The fear of becoming a fat non-smoker with no friends has little basis in reality, however, given that one can always make new friends, and post-cessation weight gain, which averages only 10 pounds, can be prevented.[48] Nonetheless, the subconscious mind may consider that remote possibility to be a real threat and prefer to maintain the "safe" status quo as a smoker. It's similar to how someone with a fear of flying might avoid air travel, although a plane crash is statistically nearly impossible.

Ask yourself how the smoking habit benefits your life and identify the drawbacks of becoming smoke-free. It's essential to consider, ahead of time, the new problems that could arise after you stop smoking and solve them so that there are no surprises. In the above example, one solution could be to increase your physical activity upon quitting and meet new people who don't smoke.

Unresolved emotional issues (especially trauma or grief)

The irrational, short-term-oriented, subconscious mind generates the emotions that drive behavior. As I explained earlier, it is usually a waste of time and energy to focus on conscious-level, willpower-dependent behavior modification when emotions are involved, as with smoking. It is possible and often easy to change subconscious programming that affects both emotion and behavior, but conventional physicians and psychotherapists are not well equipped to help you do it.

Emotional distress is an obvious and significant cause of unhealthy behavior, as compulsive behaviors like smoking provide momentary pleasure or temporary relief from discomfort, and often both.[49] Research shows that people who have serious psychological distress are more than twice as likely to smoke as those who do not.[50] Despite the conscious desire to resist this behavior, the subconscious, immediate need to avoid pain or seek pleasure usually prevails. This internal conflict explains why willpower usually fails to change habits. It also explains why some smokers who quit smoking begin overeating and gaining weight. If the emotion that drives the behavior doesn't change, a new behavior that meets the same emotional need will often replace the old behavior.

Since habitual instant gratification amounts to little more than scratching at a persistent itch, any relief or pleasure is short-lived. As a result, the behavior must be repeated until it becomes a habit. It's pointless to repeatedly scratch the "emotional itch" to eliminate stress, fear, loneliness, frustration, or sadness, because the itch is merely a symptom of the actual irritant – the disempowering thoughts, beliefs, memories, pictures, and sounds we generate and regenerate in our minds.[51]

For example, if you have a disempowering belief such as "I'm not safe," "People are always trying to cheat me," "Life is unfair," "I'm not good enough," or "It's really hard to quit smoking," you are likely to experience fear, sadness, overwhelm, or anger, which are the symptoms or effects of those thoughts or beliefs. Quite often, the beliefs that limit or damage us in the long run are intended to protect us in the short run. The belief, "I'm not safe," can cause us to feel fear and act in ways that help us avoid the risk of perceived danger, even if the belief is incorrect. Your subconscious mind has positive intentions for discouraging you from quitting smoking, including avoiding disappointment from potential failure and preventing you from abandoning a habit that has served you in so many ways for so long.

Unwanted emotional and behavioral habits are conditioned responses to learned beliefs and perceptions, which means all of them can be un-learned and deconditioned. My colleagues and I have found that the vast majority of people who suffer from obesity, panic attacks, depression, and addictions have experienced significant emotional trauma during their lifetime. Emotional trauma, including grief or loss, is also a major cause of chronic stress or anxiety. All of these issues are considered so challenging to treat largely because most treatments focus on the symptoms them-selves and ignore the underlying cause.

If you've been affected by trauma, grief, or significant anxiety, whether the origins were recent or from childhood, it's ideal to resolve it before you focus on quitting smoking. If you address only smoking and ignore the underlying issues, you're less likely to remain smoke-free.[52] The more you target the actual cause, the more thoroughly and quickly you can resolve all of the symptoms or effects, including smoking.

My wife, Gina Goodwin, and I see clients privately to resolve emo-tional trauma and its emotional and behavioral consequences. If you would like our help, visit www.GoodwinHypnosis.com to learn more.

Alcohol consumption

In my experience working with clients, alcohol consumption has been their top cause of relapse, even after they realize short-term success. The other main contributors are not using the hypnosis audios as instructed and failing to manage stress. It's common for smoking and alcohol to accom-pany each other, especially when socializing, and this page assumes that you tend to smoke when you drink. Studies show that smokers drink twice as much alcohol as nonsmokers, and alcoholism is at least four times more prevalent among those who smoke.[53,54] Drinking alcohol, either excessively or in any amount in the company of smokers, is a reliable recipe for failure in the early stages of smoking cessation.[55,56]

There are several reasons for this fact. First, alcohol impairs your judgment, so you're more likely to do something foolish after a few drinks, like light up a cigarette. Second, drinking alcohol can trigger a strong mental reminder to smoke, since the two are highly associated. Third, social pressure to drink is correlated to the social pressure to smoke, so if you're socializing with friends who do both, you're less likely to abstain from either alcohol or smoking.

It's best to avoid drinking ANY alcohol for at least a month to steer clear of any risky situations and give your brain time to reset itself chemically. After that, minimize spending time with your smoking friends whenever alcohol could be involved, just to be safe. I have found that clients who were not willing or able to abstain from alcohol for even one month were either alcoholics or just not serious about quitting smoking. That group of clients had a relatively low success rate. If you can't easily stop drinking alcohol for a month whenever you choose to do so, then it may be a good idea to address your alcohol dependency first. Feel free to contact us for help with this issue.

Looking to the Future

"The past cannot be changed. The future is yet in your power."

– Unknown

You must have something to live for.

There is an old saying, "You can't teach an old dog new tricks." Twenty-five years ago, I gained some experience training dogs, and I can tell you that this saying is wrong. Using excellent training methods along with proper motivation and rewards, I found that dogs of any age do learn new habits and unlearn old ones, no matter how long those old behaviors have been reinforced. As a hypnotist, I have gained vastly more experience as a trainer of humans, and I have found the same to be true. The main difference is that dogs' rewards (praise and food) are immediate, while the rewards for quitting smoking take days or weeks to be realized.

I realized over time that clients who were over the age of 70 had less success quitting smoking than younger clients. The number of elderly clients I saw for quitting smoking was relatively low, primarily due to the fact that most smokers quit or die before they have smoked for 50 years. Nonetheless, I saw enough to identify the common factor among successful clients – they had something inspiring or rewarding to live for. It may have been grandchildren, a good marriage, an active social life, or a career or hobby. When my clients had nothing significant to look forward to, their internal motivation was lower, so their follow-through was weaker. Younger people, even in their 50s, nearly always have more of a future to build, goals to strive for, and social and physical benefits to realize from quitting smoking.

While breaking free from the chains of smoking is its own reward, and it can be relatively easy to do so, it's still critical to have a clear idea of your expected long-term benefits from quitting smoking. What do you have to live for that inspires you? If you don't have any compelling answers, I suggest that you find them right away.

Once you are smoke-free, don't be dumb enough to start again.

Many people have sought my help to quit smoking after having returned to the mental and emotional prison of smoking following months or years of freedom. The most unfortunate example was a woman in her 70s who had been diagnosed with emphysema and referred to me by her physician. In our initial conversation, she admitted that she had smoked from age 15-30. Then on her 35th birthday, she shared with regret, she was celebrating with friends who smoked and decided to have a few cigarettes herself. Once she made it acceptable to smoke just one time, it was easier to make excuses to do it again. Within a few months, she was once again smoking one pack a day, and so it continued for another 40 years.

In other words, she had been imprisoned for 15 years and then escaped. After enjoying several years of freedom, she voluntarily chose to visit her former jailer, who promptly shackled her with chains and slammed shut the prison gates for the next 40 years.

Save yourself the regret, shame, and illness. Once you quit smoking, don't ever, ever, ever, ever do so much as touch a cigarette again, because non-smokers don't touch cigarettes. And if you need to find new friends who don't smoke, do so.

Self-Created Mental Traps

"Emancipate yourself from mental slavery.
None but ourselves can free our minds."

– Bob Marley

Living in a (dis)comfort zone

The subconscious motivation behind every cigarette you smoke is to manage your mental, emotional, or physiological state. Whether the specific urge is to alleviate discomfort, to start the day, or to calm down, the general purpose is the same. Most smokers are less tolerant of emotional discomfort than non-smokers, because they've learned to depend on a crutch to manage that discomfort. The more they smoke, the more sensitivity to discomfort they develop, and the more perceived stress they feel, the greater their desire to smoke.[57] It becomes a vicious cycle.

Do you remember the 1970s video game, Pong? Imagine a room with a paddle on each wall and a ball that is forever bouncing from one wall to the other. As long as the ball is moving through the air, everything is fine. But as the ball approaches the wall, an uncomfortable tension builds. Each time the wall paddle hits the ball, the tension is relieved and comfort returns. This is a metaphor for the smoker's comfort zone. The wall is the outer bound of the comfort zone, the ball is the smoker's mind-body state, and a paddle hitting the ball is smoking a cigarette. The more someone smokes, the smaller their comfort zone tends to be, and the faster their ball moves back and forth.

Heavy smokers are trapped in a very small comfort zone, so emotional discomfort builds quickly and easily. They smoke one upon waking, two with breakfast, another few on the drive to work, one when they get to work, one on a coffee break, a few after a phone call, some more before and after lunch, a few more with coffee in the afternoon, one after meeting with the boss, another before leaving work, a few on the drive home, one before dinner, another two after dinner, one while having a glass of wine, and then they go to sleep. Wow! That's a lot. They must smoke constantly to manage their state (whenever they're angry, happy, stressed, relaxed, hungry, full, tired, energized, bored, focused, etc.), and they feel uncomfortable when they're not smoking. You can just imagine that ball flying back and forth in their small room.

Smokers on the other end of the spectrum have a much larger comfort zone, and their ball moves more slowly. They may smoke only a few cigarettes per day, perhaps only a couple in the morning and a couple after dinner. Or maybe they smoke only while driving or before or after a stressful meeting or difficult phone call, or possibly just to unwind at the end of a workday. They can tolerate much more discomfort than a heavy smoker who has to smoke with every minor mood fluctuation or challenging situation.

The more someone depends on a substance or behavior to keep them centered, the less ability they have to center themselves without it. This fact explains the myth of the "addictive personality," which is a nonsense label applied to people who feel the need to use many substances or behaviors to balance their state. It's not a personality but an indication of how emotionally distressed those people are. Quite often, the emotional discomfort is outside of their conscious awareness, perhaps because it feels normal to them. The more emotionally uncomfortable they are, the more susceptible they are to addictive tendencies, and the more readily they will engage in compulsive behaviors. Show me an overweight gambler who drinks and smokes, and I'll show you someone with a lot of emotional pain.

Ongoing emotional discomfort can result from unresolved trauma, low self-worth, chronic stress, or lack of fulfillment. For the most part, people who have resolved their emotional baggage and are truly inspired and fulfilled in their personal and work life are nearly addiction-proof.

An effective way to eliminate addictions and compulsions is to resolve the underlying emotional distress or life dissatisfaction that makes you feel uncomfortable. What pushes you to the outer bounds of your comfort zone? How could you expand your comfort zone, so that you can stop relying on substances and compulsive habits to feel okay?

Chronic "master debating"

When one considers quitting smoking, there is usually a noticeable internal debate. You may think, "I want to stop smoking, BUT [insert your favorite excuse or fear here]." Most smokers have mastered the skill of debating (also known as bullshitting) themselves so much that they're trapped in a constant state of inner conflict. This conflict creates more stress, which then increases the urge to smoke (to alleviate the stress). As a result, the cycle of debate continues.

I've met a number of prospective clients who battled themselves at the end of our consultation when given an opportunity to proceed with my customized private session program. I call these people "master debaters." They typically admitted that they spent thousands of dollars per year on smoking, they agreed that everything I told them during our conversation made perfect sense, they had read pages and pages of my testimonials from happy ex-smokers, they believed that I could help them, and they seriously wanted to stop smoking. Once I told them the price tag, however, their subconscious mind began to fire up their insecurities – "What if it doesn't work? Can I do one session and see how it goes? Is there any guarantee? How long have you been doing this? What's your success rate? I need to ask my husband or wife or boyfriend or girlfriend or mommy or psychic or cat. Let me think about it."

The varied objections and questions were all masking the same real fear, which is that they would waste money on yet another failed attempt to quit smoking. Unfortunately, this learned expectation of failure, even among those who could easily afford it, ended up costing them much more than they bargained for.

Incidentally, I was charging as much as $1777 in 2018 when I saw my last smoking cessation client, but my fees were less than half that amount 10 years earlier. As I raised my fees, fewer people seemed to debate themselves about it, although it still happened occasionally.

I often found it humorous and pathetic how some of the master debaters who agreed to proceed often called to cancel their first session a day beforehand, citing unexpected expenses ranging from a suddenly broken air conditioning unit to an expensive car repair to a leaky roof. Couldn't they have just admitted that it wasn't worth the financial risk or that they didn't believe that they had what it took to succeed? I'm sure that their self-worth took a hit when they backed out.

I do recall one client who gave me a similar excuse after she balked at paying $977 to quit a two pack-a-day habit. She had admitted to wasting around $4,000 per year in cigarettes, not to mention all of the other tangible and intangible costs. Nonetheless, she was concerned about the price and told me that she would attempt to do it on her own, even though she had tried to quit many times over the previous 30 years. I assumed I would never hear from her again, as was often the case with master debaters. To my surprise, she contacted me five years later and said she needed my help, as she had not been able to quit on her own, and she was certain I could help her. Even though my fees had increased by $500 since our original meeting, she readily agreed to pay, as it was a minor expense after she had blown $20,000 on cigarettes in the intervening years. Ouch! I have seen many other master debaters come back to me several years and tens of thousands of dollars later.

It's important to realize that the part of the mind that generated fear and doubt in the master debaters is the same part that told them to smoke all those years. While the subconscious mind may be helpful in tending to our immediate need for self-protection, it's lousy at making long-term decisions like investing in oneself. Although it usually gives the wrong advice, most smokers are used to submissively obeying their subconscious mind's fear-based commands.

Do yourself a favor and list the various ways you debate or bullshit yourself out of great opportunities in every part of your life, including smoking, and consider what underlies your fearful objections or excuses.

Putting all of your eggs in one basket

The emotional dependency on cigarettes is directly proportional to the number or magnitude of needs that are satisfied by smoking. Why do most pack-a-day smokers have a significant emotional dependency on cigarettes? They smoke to take a work break, to relax or escape frustration, to finish a meal, to accompany wine or coffee, to socialize with friends, to distract themselves while driving, to talk on the phone, and many other situations. Someone who smokes only occasionally when drinking with friends does not meet as many emotional needs by smoking and so is less emotionally dependent on cigarettes.

The mental trap of smoking consists largely of its learned associations with so many activities, environments, and thoughts. The subconscious mind becomes so familiar with these associations that it feels uncomfortable to experience any of them without cigarettes. This is often the origin of the mistaken belief, "I need to smoke, because..." The dependency becomes so strong for many smokers that they even offer the ridiculous statement, "If I quit smoking, I wouldn't know what to do with my hands!" The fact is that non-smokers do all of those activities or handle all of those thoughts without cigarettes, and if you never taught yourself to smoke, you would do likewise.

You will discover in my quit smoking system a simple strategy for permanently eliminating the emotional dependency, so that smoking becomes a completely redundant and easily disposable behavior.

Belonging to a death cult of mental slavery

Consider someone who is lured into a secretive organization by wonderful promises of peer acceptance, exclusive social status, elevated mental or emotional states, and freedom from established authority figures. This person is then pressured by other members to engage in unsafe or harmful acts to prove his or her commitment to the group. The painful initiation process continues until the new member becomes desensitized to the discomfort, after which he or she is officially welcomed and then rewarded for joining the cult.

Membership requirements include subordinating oneself many times per day to slavishly worship the cult leader, donating thousands of dollars annually, alienating people who were important in the member's life, consuming substances that are toxic but demonstrate continued loyalty, and recruiting new members. While these requirements were not revealed to each cult member before he or she joined, most members are perfectly content to do whatever they need to do to remain in good standing.

Furthermore, the new member is repeatedly warned (even by people on the outside) how difficult it would be if he or she were to try and leave the cult, how those who attempt to escape will be punished, and how most people who actually escape do eventually return. Every year, a small percentage of members are randomly selected and ritually sacrificed against their will and without warning. More than half of all members ultimately develop an illness resulting from their involvement in this cult, and most of those people are ultimately killed off as part of their membership experience.

That sounds like a pretty awful cult, doesn't it? The government should infiltrate it, arrest its leaders, shut it down, and free and rehabilitate its enslaved members, right? Well, it's not some obscure or imaginary death cult. It's an accurate description of the lifestyle of smoking, starting with a (typically young) person being brainwashed into smoking and then becoming trapped in the habit, usually for years or decades. Brainwashing can be defined as the process of pressuring someone into adopting radically different beliefs by using systematic and often forcible means. That description definitely applies to smoking.

In the United States, smoking causes one in five deaths every year, and one in seven adults smoke cigarettes regularly, nearly half of whom have a disease caused by smoking.[58] Globally, one-fifth of adults smoke, and more than 7 million people die annually from smoking.[59] So this death cult is very powerful and widespread. Many people have escaped the cult physically, but fewer have escaped the mental slavery. To ensure your long-term health and full recovery, it is absolutely vital that you deprogram the cult's harmful belief system from your subconscious mind.

Remember Yoda's advice to Luke Skywalker: "You must unlearn what you have learned."

Part 3:
Specific Recommendations

"To think well and to consent to obey someone
giving good advice are the same thing."

– Herodotus

Emotional

It's much easier to quit smoking and stay smoke-free when you're relaxed, which is a major reason why consistent use of the hypnosis audios during the program is critical. The hypnosis sessions reprogram your thinking and recondition your nervous system to be calmer. The more relaxed you are, the easier it is to unlearn this habit, and the lower your levels of stress (a common trigger) will be.

If you have major stressors, such as a recent or still prominent traumatic experience, an ongoing hostile divorce, or a recent financial or job loss, it may be best to address those issues first. This can be done by seeing us for private sessions (www.GoodwinHypnosis.com), or by otherwise reducing your stress levels. Once you're emotionally stable and can devote your mental resources to quitting smoking, you will be ready for the program.

Social

As I explained earlier, share your goal ahead of time with a few friends who will support you. This "circle of trust" approach is usually much better than telling everyone you know or keeping it a secret. Of course, once you have completed my online program and are comfortably smoke-free, it's an excellent idea to tell anyone or everyone that you've successfully quit smoking.

Years ago, I found a study of cessation programs that reported higher long-term quit rates among those who shared their success with others, especially in writing. Consider writing down every bit of progress you make, every victory, no matter how small. And tell your friends, too!

Environmental

For at least three to four weeks following your quit date, avoid smokers (unless they live with you) and environments that you associate with smoking. Once you're comfortable and secure in your own skin as a non-smoker, then it's safe to gain some exposure to them, as long as alcohol is not involved. Remember that consuming alcohol in the presence of smokers is a recipe for disaster, especially in the first few months.

Behavioral

There are seven must-do actions as you embark on this journey:

1. Throw away ALL smoking-related items the evening before your quit day, so that you're completely smoke-free (ideally for at least 12 hours) as of your first hypnosis session.
2. Avoid consuming any alcohol for at least 30 days. If you are not willing or able do this, then you may have an alcohol dependency that should be resolved before doing my program.
3. Use my hypnosis audios as instructed, according to the schedule I provide. If you miss a session, add it to the following day's schedule. Don't cut corners or make excuses.
4. Practice the mind clearing and stress reduction exercises that come with my online system.
5. Do your best to get more sleep than usual for the first few weeks, starting before your quit day. The amount and quality of sleep you get may be associated with long-term success.[60]
6. Don't be overly concerned about your eating habits during the first week or so. Breaking the smoking habit is far more important than keeping a strict diet. Usually, any increase in sweets or snacking is temporary and can be minimized by using the hypnosis audios, the mind clearing and stress reduction exercises, and the nutritional recommendations.
7. Engage in some light to moderate physical activity for the first few weeks at a minimum. If you're not accustomed to exercising, then just do 10 minutes of brisk walking, while breathing fully,

two or three times per day. Exercise has an immediate and cumulative positive effect on brain chemistry, so this can balance any temporary dip in mood that some people experience upon quitting smoking. Research has actually found that moderate physical activity reduces cigarette cravings.[61,62] Even better, exercise will facilitate the recovery and healing of your lungs.

Nutritional

These nine dietary tips will make quitting much easier physically:

Hydration:

1. Drink at least 96 oz. of purified or distilled water throughout the day for several weeks (drink even more initially), as this will assist detoxification. Add fresh lemon or lime juice for flavor. Do not wait until you become thirsty, as thirst occurs only after you have become dehydrated.[63]
2. If you get hungry, drink a tall glass of water and take several deep breaths before eating anything, as your hunger could be thirst or stress in disguise.

Blood sugar:

3. Avoid skipping meals and make sure to eat something for breakfast. It is important to maintain a stable blood sugar level, as doing so may enhance your self-control.[64]
4. For the first several days, eat a small amount of fruit as a snack between meals. If you experience blood sugar dips or cravings for sweets, drink three or four ounces of fruit juice as needed, but start weaning off after several days. It may be more convenient to add a few ounces of juice to several 16-20 oz. bottles of water and drink them throughout the day for several days.
5. If sugar cravings are an ongoing problem for you, you may benefit from supplementing with herbs that naturally support blood sugar metabolism. Many of my clients have found Nature's Way Blood Sugar Manager to be a safe, effective, and immediate solution, either for short-term or long-term use.

Caffeine:

6. Cut caffeine intake by half immediately after your last cigarette. If you smoke only a few cigarettes per day, this step is not as important, but it's vital if you smoke at least half a pack. Do not entirely stop consuming caffeine all at once, or you may suffer headaches for several days. If you have created strong associations between drinking coffee and smoking, it may help to switch for a month to black tea, which has one-third to one-half as much caffeine per ounce.

7. If you enjoy coffee and want to eliminate or further reduce your caffeine intake, I recommend two herbal "coffees" you can make at home: Teeccino and Dandy Blend. Both mimic the coffee experience, are good for you, and taste much better than coffee.

Vegetables:

8. There is a lot of anecdotal evidence that drinking fresh vegetable juices is helpful in the weeks after your final cigarette. Some nutritionists state that raw vegetables high in chlorophyll accelerate the detoxification of nicotine and other accumulated toxins, and others say that green juices help to alkalize the smoker's acidic body. Regardless, veggies like spinach, kale, celery, and cucumber are nutritious and help to replenish a nutrient-depleted system. Buying bottles of chilled, fresh juices at the supermarket is more practical than juicing vegetables at home. Just make sure the juices are organic and have no salt, sugar, or preservatives. Many people choose a juice blend that contains apple, which makes the veggie flavor sweeter and more palatable. For variety, combine this option with tip number four on the previous page.

9. For similar reasons, it's very important to eat lots of fresh leafy greens and raw vegetables. One large, healthy salad a day can also prevent post-cessation weight gain. Just watch the dressing!

Part 4:
Frequently Asked Questions

What is hypnosis?

Hypnosis is a natural state of waking consciousness that we access automatically many times daily, most notably as we awaken and fall asleep. Everyday examples of a hypnotic state include "zoning out" while driving, daydreaming, or becoming immersed in, or emotionally responsive to, a novel, movie, or video game. All hypnosis is really self-hypnosis, so nearly everyone can experience it readily. The subconscious mind becomes more imaginative and receptive to learning and changing beliefs, perceptions, and behaviors. Hypnotic methods vary widely, so it can be difficult to evaluate hypnosis in clinical research. Nonetheless, hypnosis has been found to be quite effective for smoking cessation.[65-69]

Is hypnosis safe?

Hypnosis is completely safe for most people. It's impossible to get "stuck" in hypnosis, and you cannot be made to do anything against your will. While hypnotized, you are conscious (not asleep) and in control. The false notion that hypnosis is mind control has scared countless people away from using it for self-improvement. I have explained that the purpose of hypnosis, under the direction of a competent hypnotist, is to help you regain control of your own mind. After all, if you hadn't already lost control, you wouldn't need to see a hypnotist.

Binaural beats, an audio technology I use in my hypnosis programs to boost effectiveness, may temporarily increase the risk of seizure in epileptics. However, I've never seen a seizure nor heard any reports from clients, despite using binaural beats in over ten thousand private sessions.

Otherwise, hypnosis causes no side effects other than feeling more relaxed and sleeping better. The only warning you must respect is to avoid listening to hypnosis audios when driving or engaged in an activity that demands your full attention with your eyes open.

What is NLP?

Neurolinguistic programming, or NLP, is the practical study of how we process the information that comes from our environment and from our own thoughts. The way you think and feel about your life experiences (past, present, and future, real or imagined) affects your behavior, so changing how you process and perceive information can help you to realize your goals, such as quitting smoking, with less time and effort.

As a hypnotist, I use NLP to resolve internal conflict ("I want to quit smoking, but I keep smoking"), neutralize emotional trauma, change desire for certain foods, trigger emotional states, improve self-image or empathy, change memories, and more. Many aspects of NLP are hypnotic in that they influence the subconscious, and NLP complements hypnotism as an applied methodology for personal transformation. Blending hypnosis and NLP delivers much better results than hypnosis alone, so NLP techniques constitute an important part of my hypnosis audios.

Why should I do your program instead of seeing a hypnotist?

I believe that my system is more comprehensive and intensive than other digital quit smoking programs I have seen, and much more effective than the methods used in clinical studies. If, however, you can find a hypnotist who is skilled and experienced at smoking cessation, then he or she will be able to customize each session to your specific needs, which is not possible with a pre-designed, digital program. That being said, my program is more affordable than working privately with a hypnotist, and it has a full money back guarantee. I recommend that you use my online program first, and, if needed, consider a live hypnotist as a backup plan.

If you would like extra support, we offer a hybrid option that combines my program's digital content with live Zoom coaching sessions with me or my wife, Gina, who is also a Board Certified Hypnotist. The primary benefit of this coaching is to provide ongoing guidance, encouragement, and accountability, while also addressing any questions or challenges that may arise along the way. Visit www.GoodwinHypnosis.com to learn more about this option.

How much of a time commitment does your program require?

If you want to ensure a smooth experience and secure your long-term success, it's essential to listen to two or three hypnosis sessions per day over the 30-day period. You must carve out a few 20-30 minute blocks throughout the day when you can sit back with your eyes closed and listen without interruption. The daily time investment averages only 50 minutes, which is comparable to the total time wasted in smoking 10 cigarettes. Each of the first few days require 95 minutes, after which the required time decreases steadily to 24 minutes per day in the final week.

Before you claim that you're too busy, realize that you definitely do have time. You just need to schedule it as a higher priority than using the Internet, social media, phone, or TV. At work, you can do it in your parked car on a lunch break. In addition to helping you quit smoking, the hypnosis sessions relieve stress and can provide other unexpected benefits.

Most people quit smoking completely within the first few days, and the ones who succeed in the long run commit to the program 100% for the full 30 days, no matter how easy or difficult it may be. If you do your part, no additional time commitment or reinforcement sessions will be needed after the program ends.

Should I cut back on cigarettes in advance of my quit day?

No, it's usually better to quit smoking all at once, whether you smoke five, 15, or 40 cigarettes per day. Most of my successful clients shifted suddenly from smoking their typical amount to smoking nothing as soon as they started their hypnosis program. Research also suggests that abrupt cessation is more effective than gradual cessation, as long as other support is provided, so it is not the same as cold turkey.[70] An abrupt approach may be more effective because the biochemical adjustment period is shorter, and your attention and energy are more focused.

Quitting all at once (as with my system) is chemically the same as quitting cold turkey but very different mentally and emotionally, which is what really counts. The hypnosis component makes the experience significantly easier and vastly more effective than cold turkey.

What happens once I sign up for the program?

The day you sign up, you will gain access to a stress reduction hypnosis audio and several techniques to help you relax, clear unwanted thoughts, focus your mind, and break your emotional dependency. It's important to use these tools right away as you prepare for your quit day, which is three days later. On your quit day, and several times over the coming weeks, you'll receive a new quit smoking hypnosis audio to focus on, with directions on which to use and how frequently.

Should I use other smoking cessation aids at the same time?

First of all, it is beyond my scope of practice as a hypnotist to recommend any medication, so I will leave such recommendations to physicians and drug companies. Experience has shown me that success with my hypnosis protocol does not require the use a pharmaceutical-based cessation aid. I believe it is sufficient if you focus on using the online system and applying the knowledge in this book. While you are certainly welcome to use cessation aids during the program, I cannot in good conscience endorse the use of such drugs for several reasons.

As stated in the Introduction, nicotine replacement (patch, gum, lozenge, etc.) and prescription drugs like Zyban/Wellbutrin (bupropion) and Chantix/Champix (varenicline) have been found to have a negligible effect on long-term success rates, despite such medications outperforming placebo over 12-24 weeks.[71,72] The previous clinical studies often referenced by physicians, government agencies, and the drug companies who educate them included behavioral counseling as a key part of the intervention. At the time, the assumption was that the medications would account for most of the demonstrated effect, and that the counseling would be a relatively insignificant factor. As it turned out, the opposite was true. When the medications were since studied without counseling, there was no evidence that they improved the likelihood of cessation at one year. Other research has revealed that combining hypnosis with nicotine replacement provided results that were no better than hypnosis alone,[73] and using such products without behavioral support is no better than attempting to quit without any medication.[74]

There are two additional problems with taking smoking cessation medications while doing this program (besides their questionable effectiveness and problematic side effects).[75-77] First, compared to the 4 weeks of my program, most medications should be taken for 12-24 weeks,[78-80] so you may not feel like you've really finished, despite being smoke-free for weeks. Second, after you've succeeded, you may never know whether or not the medication was even helpful, so you could deprive yourself of the confidence boost provided by the discovery that your mind alone is powerful enough to quit smoking.

Will I gain weight after I quit smoking?

There is no reason to worry about weight gain if you use my hypnosis system and follow my recommendations, as most of my clients maintained or lost weight. Women especially tend to fear that they will gain 25-30 lbs. after quitting smoking, although that is not common. Clinical research has found that the average weight gain in the months after quitting is approximately 10 pounds, and 20% of ex-smokers actually lose weight by the end of the first year.[81] That being said, there are many things you can do to minimize or prevent weight gain once you understand what causes it.

The majority of the weight comes from the substitution of food for cigarettes, which is preventable and may occur for two reasons. One is psychological, and one is physiological. First, consuming carbohydrates or overeating makes you feel good temporarily, which was the primary motivation to smoke. This form of habit substitution rarely occurs after an effective hypnotic intervention guides the subconscious to make healthy choices. Second, as previously stated, regular nicotine intake causes artificial blood sugar spikes and suppresses appetite. As a result, quitting smoking often leads to unexpected blood sugar dips, a major symptom of which is hunger or sugar cravings (often incorrectly labeled as cigarette or nicotine cravings). This condition begins to improve after several days, as normal blood sugar management is gradually restored.

Research has also found that the act of smoking has an acute effect on metabolic rate, increasing it by up to 10% for less than 30 minutes.[82] Other research suggests that smoking may suppress the body's weight "set point" below normal levels, so quitting smoking simply restores your set point to normal.[83] This factor could lead to a gradual weight gain of a few pounds, although moderate exercise immediately upon quitting and for several weeks afterward can minimize it.

A healthy side effect of quitting smoking is a gain of one or two pounds of water due to rehydration, since many smokers are frequently dehydrated, as noted earlier. This is a positive development, because a dehydrated body doesn't burn fat efficiently, so being hydrated facilitates weight management.[84,85] Rehydration may account for one of the reasons why a number of my clients lost weight after they stopped smoking. Another reason is that their improved energy levels and lung function made exercise easier. In addition, the hypnosis sessions reduced their emotional stress, so their eating habits often improved immediately.

In summary, it's potentially easier to lose weight as a non-smoker, especially if you stay well hydrated, manage your stress, slightly improve your eating habits, and exercise moderately.

What should I do if I have cravings?

Remember that cravings are primarily emotionally driven urges that arise when the subconscious wants to do something that it's not currently doing, especially when that action conflicts with your conscious wishes. Therefore, successfully reprogramming your subconscious perception of smoking will prevent cravings from arising in the first place. If they do arise, then be sure to apply the stress reduction techniques I provide as part of my system and do your hypnosis sessions consistently.

Realize that what you consider nicotine cravings are usually adrenaline-driven cravings for sugar, food, or water, which are common short-term side effects from quitting smoking.[86] If you use my hypnosis system and follow my recommendations concerning nicotine withdrawal, any cravings will be temporary and manageable, assuming they occur at all.

If you're among the minority of readers who attempt to quit without hypnosis, rest assured that cravings typically last only a few minutes if you don't obsess about them. Here's how to handle them. Stand up, take a walk around, breathe deeply for a minute or two, and drink a glass of water, all while listening to one of your favorite feel good songs.

What happens if I slip up and have a cigarette?

The shortest path to successful cessation is to stop completely on your quit day and vow to avoid touching another cigarette. This should be your intention, focus, and commitment. Still, I have had many successful clients who smoked a few cigarettes for a couple of days after their quit day. Some reduced their intake by 80-90% before stopping completely a few days later, typically because they weren't 100% committed on their quit day. Others persisted for a few days without smoking and then had a couple of cigarettes, often because they consumed alcohol, socialized with smokers, or didn't throw away their remaining cigarettes (all of which disregarded my instructions). Both groups were also often guilty of failing to use their hypnosis programs as directed. The good news is that those who recovered by correcting their errors and recommitting to the program were almost always successful in the end.

Occasionally, clients struggle for a few weeks before quitting smoking completely. Once again, you can avoid this scenario by putting this entire book into practice and devoting your 30 days to the program. In rare cases, a person may relapse in the future (typically for reasons discussed in this book). If that happens, immediately set a new quit date, re-read this book, and repeat the entire 30-day program. You can also contact us for a private hypnosis session or enroll in the option that combines the digital content with live coaching.

Remember to avoid getting upset or blaming yourself or others if you do slip up or experience slower progress than expected. Quitting smoking is a process of relearning and retraining yourself, so stay relentlessly focused on your goal, and you will succeed.

What's your opinion on e-cigarettes and vaping?

This is a very relevant issue today, because a lot of people are shifting from smoking cigarettes to vaping electronic cigarettes. While vaping's long-term health consequences for users are currently unknown, it is likely to be less toxic than cigarettes to innocent bystanders (due to a lack of secondhand and thirdhand smoke) and may even be less dangerous to users. Still, I encourage you quit completely, as opposed to switching to vaping.

Cigarette manufacturers' long-term business strategy is to shift from selling conventional cigarettes to e-cigarettes, a transition that will likely benefit public health. On an individual basis, however, vaping is still very unhealthy mentally and behaviorally, because users remain emotionally dependent on their habit. Consider that most smokers are acutely aware of the physiological impact, smell, inconvenience, social stigma, and expense associated with smoking, while the only obvious disadvantage of vaping is its greater financial cost. Unfortunately, when a smoker shifts to e-cigarettes, he or she loses nearly all of the discomfort, hassle, and negativity once associated with smoking cigarettes, so he or she loses significant motivation to quit completely.

Don't rob yourself of the opportunity to make use of this mental pain, disgust, and frustration from smoking cigarettes. Take full advantage of it to help you quit altogether. I believe that our society will eventually be free of cigarettes, but the percentage of people who vape may be much higher than those who currently smoke cigarettes. The quit rate will be much lower because vaping is more acceptable and convenient. The tobacco companies are expecting you to fall into this trap – you think you're doing something better for yourself by switching to e-cigarettes, and then they know you have become a customer for life.

Send your subconscious mind a clear message that you're a nicotine-free non-smoker by staying away from any unhealthy substitutes like e-cigarettes. And if you currently smoke and vape, it's best to quit both at the same time.

Conclusion

"One can choose to go back toward safety or forward toward growth.
Growth must be chosen again and again; fear must be overcome again and again."

– Abraham Maslow

Congratulations on completing this book! By now, you have a much broader and deeper understanding of smoking cessation from a mental, emotional, and physiological perspective. Moreover, you possess more accurate, relevant, and actionable knowledge on this topic than do many doctors, therapists, nutritionists, hypnotists, and any of your friends.

That being said, knowledge is not power. It's only potential power. You must act on your knowledge to benefit from it, or else this book will have served only as intellectual entertainment. Realize that no one can make you quit smoking. Only you can decide to do it because you want to do it.

Here is a quick review of the key points:

- Quit making excuses if you want to quit smoking.
- Don't waste time hoping that you'll succeed.
- Do or do not. There is no try.
- Don't wait for a medical warning or emergency to quit.
- Reflect upon the death cult of mental slavery and consider if you are really ready to discontinue your membership.
- Consider how your life will improve once you're smoke-free.
- Stop debating yourself and take action.
- Find other ways to satisfy the needs you met by smoking.
- Consider how your relationships could sabotage you and share your goal only with those who will support your efforts.
- Pay for the online hypnosis system yourself, focus relentlessly on your goal, and commit 100% to completing the full program.
- Remember what causes nicotine withdrawal symptoms and manage your hydration, caffeine, and blood sugar levels accordingly.

- Manage your stress and other emotional issues.
- Expand your comfort zone.
- Get plenty of sleep and increase your physical activity.
- Avoid smokers for several weeks after your quit day.
- Beware of alcohol as one of the greatest threats to your success.
- Once you've quit smoking, vow never to touch a cigarette again.

I encourage you to re-read this book several times during the first few weeks and take notes on whatever resonates with you. As you do so, you will notice details that you didn't see the first time. Assuming you fully apply the knowledge that I've shared with you while you use my online hypnosis system, it's likely that you will succeed more easily and naturally than most people you know.

This is your moment to right all of the wrongs you have committed against your mind and body throughout the years. You need to earn your freedom, so this process must be your top priority for the first few weeks after your quit day. Give this time to yourself. You deserve it.

I have found that some people quit smoking for a short time merely by reading this book. To firmly embed that change and ensure that this is the last time you ever need to quit smoking, sign up today for my hypnosis system at www.BreakTheChainsOfSmoking.com/hypnosis. The money back guarantee will give you the confidence to take action right away.

You will never have to worry about smoking again if you do this properly. Give your greatest commitment as you reclaim your freedom and begin your journey home to your new life as a non-smoker. Your future self will thank you.

I look forward to hearing about your success!

More Client Testimonials

"I worked with Todd many years ago and I am living proof that it works. I had a nasty cigarette habit - I am European, that sums it all!! I would quit and even a year later slowly start again, at a party after a glass of wine it was always a perfect excuse to smoke "only one" ---- the one turned me quickly into a smoker again! The dreams, the nightmares, the anxiety, the yearning for that smoke made it all very hard for me to stay clean! Well almost 7 years ago on Valentines day, I went to see Todd and after the first session I was free of it! I have never smoked again, never had dreams, never suffered any of the withdrawal symptoms of stopping this ugly smelly harsh addiction. He taught me several other things to use in my daily life because he is very knowledgeable and helpful. He is awesome and really cares!!! Thank you Todd!!"

– Helena G.

"There are no amount of words, no amount of anything to express the gratitude I give daily for having stumbled across the expeditious and wonderful life transforming miracle that is hypnosis with Todd Goodwin."

– Jessica Dolores

"I always smoked when drinking, hanging out with friends after work in South Beach or doing anything social. I was afraid I'd have to give all that up, but now I have more fun not feeling like I have to smoke all the time. Because of my decision to stop smoking and the support of your hypnosis services, my social life has improved a lot. It's so much easier to meet new people and make new friends now that I don't smoke anymore. I'm going to keep referring my smoking buddies to you so all of them can stop smoking, too."

– Ricky Rodriguez

"I think Todd's method is the most effective from any others I tried and what is the most important - you can feel he really cares about you and the result you are getting!"

– Anna

"As a single mom, I was under a lot of stress from work and my family life, having to juggle so many things. All I can say is WOW! You have taught me so much more than learning to relax, like how to clear my mind of worry and fear. What a transformation! Thank you so much!"

– Kathy Ramirez

"Todd Goodwin is seriously the best. Great experience, highly recommend it!"

– Evelyn Mendal

"I was skeptical and didn't really understand what it was. In ways I still don't understand because it is so unbelievable how something so easy to do could fix what seemed totally impossible. It is truly amazing how effective and well this worked. Looking back, it feels like a flick of a switch. Maybe it won't happen as fast for everyone but it really truly works. This completely changed my life and I'm so grateful for it. Its so simple and effortless it almost doesn't seem real. This is the best investment I have ever made and will recommend this to everybody. I have such gratitude Todd and his practice because I feel like I am back to the person I'm supposed to be."

– Oscar N.

"You have a gift. How grateful I am to be able to get a taste of it. Thank you."

– Julie Jacko

"I can tell you that Todd Goodwin really knows what he is doing. I think what impressed me the most about Todd was how he truly cares about the wellbeing and life improvement of his Client's. Thanks again Todd!!"

– Jared Shapiro

"My sessions with Todd planted seeds for self improvement that continue to grow daily and I can say that my investment in hypnotherapy was worth every penny. Todd strives to be the best at his profession and from what I can tell, he is. 5 Stars all the way!"

– Alex B.

"Todd makes this work less "painful" than most therapists I've seen, mostly because he knows when to go deep and when to make you smile and you can truly feel how much he loves what he does. Thank you for everything you offer and the authenticity with which you do your work. It shows."

– Alison Lessard

"Thank you so much for everything that you've done! Your support and expertise have made such a tremendous impact on my life and I'm so grateful that the Universe connected us."

– Alex Martel

"Fantastic experience! I highly recommend Todd Goodwin. The man is a very passionate and forward thinking professional who helped me look past my deepest insecurities, and into the abundance mentality that has changed my life in all fields. A true master of self actualization!"

– Chris Reyes

"I was able to release a lot of what was holding me back. It is truly amazing how the subconscious part of our minds rules every other aspect of our lives. Todd is not only effective, but committed, caring, and most of all, extremely professional and a master of his craft."

– Osmara Vindel

"I felt the difference in my actions and thoughts within one day. What I love about Todd the most is his ability to make you feel at ease and make you feel like you're not crazy."

– Nikki Novo

"Todd: Quick note....I have not had the DESIRE for a cigarette since I left your office. You are a very gifted person and you continue to change my life. If there is anything I can ever do to let the world know of your incredible dedication and talent to the improvement of the quality of your clients' lives, please know that you can completely count on me. God bless you always."

– Alina

The above comments were made by former clients of Todd Goodwin and are true and factual. The author does not imply or claim that these comments represent typical results. Results vary depending on age, gender, lifestyle, motivation, and individual commitment to achieve a desired result. These clients voluntarily offered their written feedback and were not compensated in any way. Each comment and/or testimonial is the opinion of one person at a specific time and should only be considered in that context.

References

1. Baker TB, Piper ME, Stein JH, et al. (2016). Effects of Nicotine Patch vs. Varenicline vs. Combination Nicotine Replacement Therapy on Smoking Cessation at 26 Weeks: A Randomized Clinical Trial. *JAMA;315*(4):371-379.

2. Leas EC, Pierce JP, Benmarhnia T, White MM, Noble ML, Trinidad DR, Strong DR. (2017). Effectiveness of Pharmaceutical Smoking Cessation Aids in a Nationally Representative Cohort of American Smokers. *JNCI: Journal of the National Cancer Institute;110*(6):581–587.

3. Hughes JR, Keely J, Naud S. (2004). Shape of the Relapse Curve and Long-Term Abstinence Among Untreated Smokers. *Addiction;99*(1):29-38.

4. Doran CM, Valenti L, Robinson M, Britt H, Mattick RP. (2006). Smoking Status of Australian General Practice Patients and Their Attempts to Quit. *Addictive Behaviors;31*(5):758-766.

5. Zhu SH, Cummins S, Gamst A, Wong S, Ikeda T. (2016). Quitting Smoking Before and After Varenicline: A Population Study Based on Two Representative Samples of US Smokers. *Tobacco Control;25*(4):464-469.

6. Kodirov SA. (2017). Addictive Neurons. *Therapeutic Targets for Neurological Diseases; 4*: e1498.

7. Stead LF, Perera R, Bullen C, Mant D, Lancaster T. (2008). Nicotine Replacement Therapy for Smoking Cessation. *Cochrane Database Syst Rev;23;*(1):CD000146.

8. Pierce JP, Gilpin EA. (2002). Impact of Over-the-Counter Sales on Effectiveness of Pharmaceutical Aids for Smoking Cessation. *JAMA;288*(10):1260-1264.

9. Hughes JR, Shiffman S, Callas P, Zhang J. (2003). A Meta-Analysis of the Efficacy of Over-the-Counter Nicotine Replacement. *Tobacco Control;12*(1):21–27.

10. Baumeister RF, Vohs KD, Tice DM. (2007). The Strength Model of Self-Control. *Current Directions in Psychological Science;16*(6): 351-355.

11. Gailliot MT, Baumeister RF, DeWall CN, Maner JK, Plant EA, Tice DM, Brewer LE, Schmeichel BJ. (2007). Self-Control Relies on Glucose as a Limited Energy Source: Willpower is More Than a Metaphor. *Journal of Personality and Social Psychology;92*;(2):325-336.

12. Tice, DM, Baumeister RF, Shmueli D, Muraven M. (2007). Restoring the Self: Positive Affect Helps Improve Self-Regulation Following Ego Depletion. *Journal of Experimental Social Psychology;43*(3):379-384.

13. Fagerstrom K. (2014). Nicotine: Pharmacology, Toxicity and Therapeutic Use. *Journal of Smoking Cessation;9*(2):53–59.

14. Maddatu J, Anderson-Baucum E, Evans-Molina C. (2017). Smoking and the Risk of Type 2 Diabetes. *Translational Research;184*:101-107.

15. Ponciano-Rodriguez G, Paez-Martinez N, Villa-Romero A, Gutierrez-Grobe Y, Mendez-Sanchez N. (2014). Early Changes in the Components of the Metabolic Syndrome in a Group of Smokers after Tobacco Cessation. *Metabolic Syndrome and Related Disorders;12*(4):242-50.

16. Parsons WD, Neims AH. (1978). Effect of Smoking on Caffeine Clearance. *Clinical Pharmacology & Therapeutics;24*(1):40-5.

17. Moore PJ, Reidel B, Ghosh A, Sesma J, Kesimer M, Tarran R. (2018). Cigarette Smoke Modifies and Inactivates SPLUNC1, Leading to Airway Dehydration. *The FASEB Journal;32*(12):6559–6574.

18. Salz A. (2014). Substance Abuse and Nutrition. *Today's Dietitian;16*(12):44.

19. Helliker K. Nicotine Fix - Behind Antismoking Policy, Influence of Drug Industry. *Wall Street Journal;* Feb 28, 2007. https://whyquit.com/nrt/wsj_helliker_nicotine_fix_020807.html

20. McLaughlin I, Dani JA, De Biasi M. (2015). Nicotine Withdrawal. *Current Topics in Behavioral Neurosciences;*24:99–123.

21. Nordqvist C. (2019). All About Hypoglycemia (Low Blood Sugar). https://www.medicalnewstoday.com/articles/166815.php

22. Kaplan GB, Greenblatt DJ, Ehrenberg BL, Goddard JE, Cotreau MM, Harmatz JS, Shader RI. (1997). Dose-Dependent Pharmacokinetics and Psychomotor Effects of Caffeine in Humans. *Journal of Clinical Pharmacology;37*:693–703.

23. Benelam B, Wyness L. (2010). Hydration and Health: A Review. *Nutrition Bulletin;35*(1):3-25.

24. Salz A. (2014). Substance Abuse and Nutrition. *Today's Dietitian;16*(12):44.

25. Morgan TM, Crawford L, Stoller A, Toth D, Yeo KT, Baron JA. (2004). Acute Effects of Nicotine on Serum Glucose Insulin Growth Hormone and Cortisol in Healthy Smokers. *Metabolism;53*(5):578-82.

26. Jessen A, Buemann B, Toubro S, Skovgaard IM, Astrup A. (2005). The Appetite-Suppressant Effect of Nicotine is Enhanced by Caffeine. *Diabetes, Obesity and Metabolism;7*(4):327-33.

27. Śliwińska-Mossoń M, Milnerowicz H. (2017). The Impact of Smoking on the Development of Diabetes and Its Complications. *Diabetes & Vascular Disease Research;14*(4)265–276.

28. Bajaj M. (2012). Nicotine and Insulin Resistance: When the Smoke Clears. *Diabetes;61*(12):3078-3080.

29. West R, Courts S, Beharry S, May S, Hajek P. (1999). Acute Effect of Glucose Tablets on Desire to Smoke. *Psychopharmacology;147*(3): 319–321.

30. McRobbie H, Hajek P. (2004). Effect of Glucose on Tobacco Withdrawal Symptoms in Recent Quitters Using Bupropion or Nicotine Replacement. *Human Psychopharmacology: Clinical & Experimental;19*(1):57-61.

31. West R, Willis N. (1998). Double-Blind Placebo Controlled Trial of Dextrose Tablets and Nicotine Patch in Smoking Cessation. *Psychopharmacology;136*(2):201–204.

32. Parsons WD, Neims AH. (1978). Effect of Smoking on Caffeine Clearance. *Clinical Pharmacology & Therapeutics;24*(1):40-5.

33. Benowitz NL, Hall SM. (1989). Persistent Increase in Caffeine Concentrations in People Who Stop Smoking. *BMJ;298*:1075.

34. de Leon J, Diaz FJ, Rogers T, Browne D, Dinsmore L, Ghosheh OH, Dwoskin LP, Crooks PA. (2003). A Pilot Study of Plasma Caffeine Concentrations in a US Sample of Smoker and Nonsmoker Volunteers. *Progress in Neuro-Psychopharmacology & Biological Psychiatry; 27*(1):165-71.

35. Bjørngaard JH, Nordestgaard AT, Taylor AE, Treur JL, Gabrielsen ME, Munafò MR, Nordestgaard BG, Åsvold BO, Romundstad P, Davey Smith G. (2017). Heavier Smoking Increases Coffee Consumption: Findings from a Mendelian Randomization Analysis. *International Journal of Epidemiology;46*(6):1958-1967.

36. Swanson JA, Lee JW, Hopp JW, Berk LS. (1997). The Impact of Caffeine Use on Tobacco Cessation and Withdrawal. *Addictive Behaviors;22*(1):55-68.

37. Curatolo PW, Robertson D. (1983). The Health Consequences of Caffeine. *Annals of Internal Medicine;98*(5 Pt 1):641-53.

38. Moore PJ, Reidel B, Ghosh A, Sesma J, Kesimer M, Tarran R. (2018). Cigarette Smoke Modifies and Inactivates SPLUNC1, Leading to Airway Dehydration. *The FASEB Journal;32*(12):6559–6574.

39. Kruszelnicki K. (2019). Why Does Drinking Alcohol Cause Dehydration? http://www.abc.net.au/science/articles/2012/02/28/3441707.htm

40. Britt JP, Bonci A. (2013). Alcohol and Tobacco: How Smoking May Promote Excessive Drinking. *Neuron;79*(3):406–407.

41. Salz A. (2014). Substance Abuse and Nutrition. *Today's Dietitian;16*(12):44.

42. WalletHub. (2018). The Real Cost of Smoking by State. https://wallethub.com/edu/the-financial-cost-of-smoking-by-state/9520/

43. McKee SA, Sinha R, Weinberger AH, Sofuoglu M, Harrison ELR, Lavery M, Wanzer J. (2010). Stress Decreases the Ability to Resist Smoking and Potentiates Smoking Intensity and Reward. *Journal of Psychopharmacology;25*(4)490-502.

44. Wang TW, Asman K, Gentzke AS, et al. (2018). Tobacco Product Use Among Adults—United States, 2017. *Morbidity and Mortality Weekly Report;67*(44):1225-32

45. U.S. Department of Health and Human Services, Centers for Disease Control and Prevention. Fast Facts. https://www.cdc.gov/tobacco/data_statistics/fact_sheets/fast_facts/

46. The Ontario Tobacco Survey. https://www.otru.org/projects/cessation/ots-technical-documentation

47. Goodwin GM. (2017). Secondary Gain.

48. Aubin HJ, Aveyard P, Farley A, Lahmek P, Lycett D. (2012). Weight Gain in Smokers After Quitting Cigarettes: Meta-Analysis. *BMJ;345*:e4439

49. Goodwin TD. (2019). Don't Get Lost in the Weeds, Uproot Them!

50. Wang TW, Asman K, Gentzke AS, et al. (2018). Tobacco Product Use Among Adults—United States, 2017. *Morbidity and Mortality Weekly Report;67*(44):1225-32.

51. Goodwin TD. (2019). Don't Get Lost in the Weeds, Uproot Them!

52. Augustson EM, Wanke KL, Rogers S, Bergen AW, Chatterjee N, Snyder K, Albanes D, Taylor PR, Caporaso NE. (2008). Predictors of Sustained Smoking

Cessation: A Prospective Analysis of Chronic Smokers From the Alpha-Tocopherol Beta-Carotene Cancer Prevention Study. *American Journal of Public Health;* 98(3): 549–555.

53. Grant BF, Hasin DS, Chou SP, Stinson FS, Dawson DA. (2004). Nicotine Dependence and Psychiatric Disorders in the United States: Results From the National Epidemiologic Survey on Alcohol and Related Conditions. *Archives of General Psychiatry;61*(11):1107-1115.

54. Larsson A, Engel JA. (2004). Neurochemical and Behavioral Studies on Eethanol and Nicotine Interactions. *Neuroscience & Biobehavioral Reviews;27*(8):713-20.

55. Augustson EM, Wanke KL, Rogers S, Bergen AW, Chatterjee N, Snyder K, Albanes D, Taylor PR, Caporaso NE. (2008). Predictors of Sustained Smoking Cessation: A Prospective Analysis of Chronic Smokers From the Alpha-Tocopherol Beta-Carotene Cancer Prevention Study. *American Journal of Public Health;* 98(3): 549–555.

56. Lynch KL, Twesten JE, Stern A, Augustson EM. (2018). Level of Alcohol Consumption and Successful Smoking Cessation. *Nicotine & Tobacco Research;nty142.*

57. Childs E, de Wit H. (2010). Effects of Acute Psychosocial Stress on Cigarette Craving and Smoking. *Nicotine & Tobacco Research;12*(4):449-453.

58. U.S. Department of Health and Human Services, Centers for Disease Control and Prevention, National Center for Chronic Disease Prevention and Health Promotion, Office on Smoking and Health. (2014). *The Health Consequences of Smoking—50 Years of Progress: A Report of the Surgeon General.*

59. World Health Organization. (2017). *WHO Report on the Global Tobacco Epidemic, External.*

60. Patterson F, Grandner MA, Malone SK, Rizzo A, Davey A, Edwards DG. (2019). Sleep as a Target for Optimized Response to Smoking Cessation Treatment. *Nicotine & Tobacco Research;21*(2): 139–148.

61. Haasova M, Warren FC, Ussher M, Van Rensburg KJ, Faulkner G, Cropley M, Byron-Daniel J, Everson-Hock ES, Oh H, Taylor AH. (2013). The Acute Effects of Physical Activity on Cigarette Cravings: Systematic Review and Meta-Analysis with Individual Participant Data. *Addiction;108*(1):26-37.

62. Scerbo F, Faulkner G, Taylor A, Thomas S. (2010). Effects of Exercise on Cravings to Smoke: The Role of Exercise Intensity and Cortisol. *Journal of Sports Sciences;28*(1):11-19.

63. Armstrong LE. (2005). Hydration Assessment Techniques. *Nutrition Reviews;63*:S40–S54.

64. Gailliot MT, Baumeister RF, DeWall CN, Maner JK, Plant EA, Tice DM, Brewer LE, Schmeichel BJ. (2007). Self-Control Relies on Glucose as a Limited Energy Source: Willpower is More Than a Metaphor. *Journal of Personality and Social Psychology;92*;(2):325-336.

65. Viswesvaran C, Schmidt FL. (1992). A Meta-Analytic Comparison of the Effectiveness of Smoking Cessation Methods. *Journal of Applied Psychology;77*(4):554-561.

66. Elkins G, Marcus J, Bates J, Rajab MH, Cook T. (2006). Intensive Hypnotherapy for Smoking Cessation: A Prospective Study. *International Journal of Clinical and Experimental Hypnosis;54*(3):303-315.

67. Tahiri M, Mottillo S, Joseph L, Pilote L, Eisenberg MJ. (2012). Alternative Smoking Cessation Aids: A Meta-analysis of Randomized Controlled Trials. *The American Journal of Medicine;125*(6):576-584.

68. Johnson DL, Karkut RT. (1994). Performance by Gender in a Stop-Smoking Program Combining Hypnosis and Aversion. *Psychological Reports;75*(2):851-7.

69. Green JP, Lynn SJ. (2000). Hypnosis and Suggestion-Based Approaches to Smoking Cessation: An Examination of the Evidence. *International Journal of Clinical and Experimental Hypnosis;48*(2):195-224.

70. Lindson-Hawley N, Banting M, West R, Michie S, Shinkins B, Aveyard P. (2016). Gradual Versus Abrupt Smoking Cessation: A Randomized, Controlled Noninferiority Trial. *Annals of Internal Medicine;164*(9):585-592.

71. Baker TB, Piper ME, Stein JH, et al. (2016). Effects of Nicotine Patch vs. Varenicline vs. Combination Nicotine Replacement Therapy on Smoking Cessation at 26 Weeks: A Randomized Clinical Trial. *JAMA;315*(4):371-379.

72. Leas EC, Pierce JP, Benmarhnia T, White MM, Noble ML, Trinidad DR, Strong DR. (2017). Effectiveness of Pharmaceutical Smoking Cessation Aids in a Nationally Representative Cohort of American Smokers. *JNCI: Journal of the National Cancer Institute;110*(6):581–587.

73. Hasan FM, Zagarins SE, Pischke KM, Saiyed S, Bettencourt AM, Beal L, Macys D, Aurora S, McCleary N. (2014). Hypnotherapy is More Effective Than

Nicotine Replacement Therapy for Smoking Cessation: Results of a Randomized Controlled Trial. *Complementary Therapies in Medicine;22*(1):1-8.

74. Kotz D, Brown J, West R. (2014). 'Real-World' Effectiveness of Smoking Cessation Treatments: A Population Study. *Addiction;*109(3):491-9.

75. Wellbutrin Side Effects.
https://www.rxlist.com/wellbutrin-side-effects-drug-center.htm

76. Chantix Side Effects.
https://www.rxlist.com/chantix-side-effects-drug-center.htm

77. Mills EJ, Wu P, Lockhart I, Wilson K, Ebbert JO. Adverse Events Associated with Nicotine Replacement Therapy (NRT) for Smoking Cessation. A Systematic Review and Meta-Analysis of One Hundred and Twenty Studies Involving 177,390 Individuals. *Tobacco Induced Diseases;8*(1):8.

78. Three Ways To Quit.
https://www.chantix.com/getting-started-with-chantix/three-ways-to-quit

79. Nicotine Replacement Therapy for Quitting Tobacco.
https://www.cancer.org/healthy/stay-away-from-tobacco/guide-quitting-smoking/nicotine-replacement-therapy.html

80. Zyban Prescribing Information.
https://www.gsksource.com/pharma/content/dam/GlaxoSmithKline/US/en/Prescribing_Information/Zyban/pdf/ZYBAN-PI-MG.PDF

81. Aubin HJ, Aveyard P, Farley A, Lahmek P, Lycett D. (2012). Weight Gain in Smokers After Quitting Cigarettes: Meta-Analysis. *BMJ;345*:e4439

82. Perkins KA. (1992). Metabolic Effects of Cigarette Smoking. *Journal of Applied Physiology;72*(2):401-9.

83. Perkins KA. (1993). Weight Gain Following Smoking Cessation. *Journal of Consulting and Clinical Psychology;61*(5):768-77.

84. Thornton SN. (2016). Increased Hydration Can Be Associated with Weight Loss. *Frontiers in Nutrition;10*(3):18.

85. Keller U, Szinnai G, Bilz S, Berneis K. (2003). Effects of Changes in Hydration on Protein, Glucose and Lipid Metabolism in Man: Impact on Health. *European Journal of Clinical Nutrition;57*;Suppl 2:S69-74.

86. Salz A. (2014). Substance Abuse and Nutrition. *Today's Dietitian;16*(12):44.

Made in the USA
Coppell, TX
06 November 2023

23869113R00050